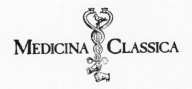

Medicina Classica

SURGICAL INSTRUMENTS
IN GREEK AND ROMAN TIMES

SURGICAL INSTRUMENTS
IN GREEK AND ROMAN TIMES

BY

JOHN STEWART MILNE, M.A., M.D. Aberd.

KEITH GOLD MEDALLIST IN CLINICAL SURGERY

WITH ILLUSTRATIONS

Augustus M. Kelley · Publishers

NEW YORK 1970

First Published 1907
(London: At The Clarendon Press)

Reprinted 1970 By
AUGUSTUS M. KELLEY, PUBLISHERS
NEW YORK, NEW YORK 10001

By Arrangement with
OXFORD UNIVERSITY PRESS

SBN 678 03755 8
Library of Congress Catalogue Card Number
70-95630

Printed in the United States of America

PREFACE

THE object of this book is to lay before the student of medical history an account of the various instruments with which the ancient Greek and Roman surgeons prosecuted their craft. It is self-evident that no clear conception of a surgical operation, ancient or modern, can be formed from a written description without some previous knowledge of the instruments intended to be used. Many interesting operations described in detail in the classical authors are rendered obscure or quite unintelligible from lack of this knowledge. The learned Adams gives an accurate translation of a long and involved chapter by Paulus Aegineta on the use of the vaginal speculum, but remarks that owing to our want of knowledge of the specula possessed by the ancients the chapter is unintelligible. Daremberg says it is impossible to say what was the shape of any of the cutting instruments mentioned by Hippocrates. The steady progress of archaeological discovery has gradually added find after find of surgical instruments, till now there is scarcely a museum with any considerable number of antique *petits bronzes* which does not number among its contents a few surgical instruments, and in the Naples Museum alone there are hundreds. In several cases we know even the name of the original possessor of these and the special branch of surgery which he practised. There are thus open to us materials which were not available to the men of learning to whom I have referred above, and the time seems opportune to undertake a systematic review of all the materials at our disposal, and attempt to reconstruct the surgical armamentarium of the ancients. Considering the importance of the subject, it is surprising that no such systematic attempt has previously

been made. Indeed, comparatively little attention has
been given to this department of archaeology. Literature
bearing on it is comparatively scarce. What we have is
entirely continental, and consists of a series of reports of
different finds with attempts to indicate the uses of the
instruments described. In addition to these reports and
the actual instruments scattered over various museums, we
have at our disposal the writings of the ancient authors
themselves. In these a fair number of instruments are
minutely described, while many others are named, and here
and there points about their shape are mentioned in different
places; and by piecing these particulars together and deduc-
ing other facts from the nature of the manipulations the
instruments are employed in, we can describe in detail, with
a tolerable amount of certainty, a surprisingly large number
of instruments. It must be confessed that these ancient
classics are rather difficult of access, surprisingly so considering that until a few decades ago they were reverenced
as works of authority for medical practice; but the fact seems
to be that our predecessors were largely content to draw
their knowledge of these authors from mediaeval Latin
translations. Part of one of the most interesting authors
has never been published in the original Greek, and for our
knowledge of it we are dependent on a sixteenth-century
Latin translation, supplemented, it may be, by fugitive
consultations of codices in libraries and museums.

Others of the Greek texts have not been reprinted
since the sixteenth century, and bristle with the ingenious
but at first perplexing shorthand contractions with which
the Renaissance typographer imitated the Compendia of
the manuscripts. These difficulties can be got over with
patience, however, and the waste of gray matter necessary
as a preliminary is not out of proportion to the results to be
obtained. Even as a quarry for philological materials the
medical classics are far from being worked out, and it is
surprising how many words one meets with which are not
to be found in the best Greek-English dictionaries.

The method pursued in the present investigation was to make a complete examination of the classical medical, surgical, anatomical, and pharmaceutical writings which have been preserved to us, copying out the portions in which an instrument was mentioned. These extracts were then rearranged in ledger form, each extract being classified under the heading of the instrument it referred to. Out of the enormous number of references thus obtained, those passages were selected which seemed to throw any light on the shape and size of the instrument to which they referred. Next, an examination was made of the reports of finds in various localities; as many specimens in various museums were examined as possible; and annotations of classical texts were searched for any further information they might give. The total information thus gained is so arranged that under the heading of each instrument will be found a series of selected extracts from different authors, with the deductions from them which it is possible to make regarding the appearance of the instrument, and an illustration is given of it from some ancient specimen where such is in existence. Failing actual ancient specimens, I have fallen back on mediaeval or ancient Arabian authors for illustration.

I have omitted a discussion of the many interesting mechanical contrivances for the reduction of deformities due to fracture and dislocation, and also of the splints, pads, and bandages for maintaining these injuries in position. These form such a well-defined group that they might fitly form the subject of a special monograph, and the illustrations required are of a different nature from those in the present volume. The majority of these contrivances will be found described in a chapter by Heliodorus preserved in Oribasius. I have omitted also all reference to the numerous forms of vessels in which the ancients prepared and stored their medicaments, with the exception of those which are intended for carrying on the person. Some of these merge into forms which are common to both drug and instrument cases, and it is impossible to separate them. It has been necessary also to include as far as possible the instruments involved in the preparation and application of medicaments, as most of these are either actually or potentially implements of minor surgery.

The volume opens with a short account of the ancient authors whose writings have any bearing on the subject in hand. At the end of the book will be found a bibliography of reports on finds, and a list of the most interesting instruments to be found in various museums. The latter makes no pretence of being a complete inventory, although it might serve as a skeleton for the construction of a more comprehensive list at some future date. The bibliography, on the other hand, is believed to be fairly complete. The bulk of the book consists of an attempt to reconstruct, in the manner described above, the different instruments used in classical times.

The books from which I have drawn most information are Brunner's *Die Spuren der römischen Ärzte auf dem Boden der Schweiz*, Deneffe's *Étude sur la Trousse d'un Chirurgien Gallo-Romain du IIIe Siècle*, Adams' translation of Paulus Aegineta, and the papers of Vulpes in the volume for 1851 of the *Memorie della Regale Accademia Ercolanese di Archeologia*.

During the five or six years which I have spent on this investigation I have unsparingly laid all my friends under contribution whenever opportunity occurred; but among those to whom I am particularly indebted I may mention Mr. M. G. Swallow of Baden, who has given me much assistance in working up the Swiss finds, Professor Alexander Ogston, under whom I spent many happy days as house-surgeon, and who has all along kept a fatherly eye on the progress of the work and encouraged me to proceed to the end with a task which at times seemed inclined to swamp me, Mr. R. C. Bosanquet, late director of the British Archaeological School at Athens, who procured for me photographs of the instruments in the Athens museum, and Mr. H. R. Nielsen of Hartlepool, who has been the companion of my wanderings among the continental museums. I have also to thank my father, John Milne, LL.D., for much help at many different points.

The expense of visiting the museums in the North of France and of obtaining photographs of the instruments in them has been borne by a grant from the Carnegie University Research Fund.

This monograph was presented as the thesis which forms part of the examination for the degree of M.D. of the University of Aberdeen, and it was successful in gaining ' Highest Honours.'

HARTLEPOOL,
April 19, 1907.

CONTENTS

CHAPTER I

INTRODUCTORY

THE earliest classical writer on medical subjects is Hippocrates, who was born in 460 B. C. and who practised in Athens
and other parts of Greece. The 'Hippocratic Collection'
is well known to consist of works which are not all by
Hippocrates himself, but as the pseudo-Hippocratic works
all belong to the classical period they are all admissible
as evidence for our purpose, and for the sake of brevity
I shall throughout refer to them as if all were by Hippocrates. Many interesting instruments are named in the
comparatively small collection of treatises which make up
the admittedly genuine list of Hippocratic works, but, taking
these along with the pseudo-Hippocratic works, the number
of instruments named in the whole collection is surprisingly
large, comprising as it does trephines, bone drills, probes,
needles, tooth forceps, uvula forceps, bone elevators, uterine
sounds, graduated dilators, cranioclasts, and others. After
Hippocrates there is a break in the continuity of the
literature, and for some hundreds of years Greek medicine is represented almost entirely by the Alexandrian
Schools. The first printed edition of the Hippocratic
works was a Latin translation printed at Rome in 1525,
followed by the Aldine edition of the Greek text printed
at Venice in the following year. Other editions are the
edition of Föes (1595), Van der Linden (1665), Kühn
(Leipzig, 1821). Later editions are the text with a French
translation by Littré (10 vols., 1849–61), a scholarly

edition by Ermerins with a Latin rendering (1859–64), and an excellent translation of the genuine works of Hippocrates by the world-famous Dr. Adams of Banchory (Sydenham Soc. Trans., 1849). The best edition, however, is the edition of Kuehlewein, begun in 1894 and at present in course of publication by Teubner, Leipzig. The later volumes have not yet appeared. For the portion of the text which is not contained in the first two volumes of Kuehlewein I have relied on the edition of Kühn for most of the readings, although occasionally those of Van der Linden or Föes are to be preferred. The references given are to the volumes and pages of Kühn's edition, but in this edition indications are given of the corresponding localities in the other editions so that cross-references to these can easily be made. There seems to be a different arrangement in different editions of Föes, for Liddell and Scott say the references in their Lexicon are to the pages in Föes but they do not correspond in any way to the pagination of the edition before me (Frankfort, 1595).

Aulus Cornelius Celsus is the next writer we have. His system of medicine in eight books is a marvel of lucid arrangement, and his beautiful style makes it a pleasure to read any of his works. The seventh book gives a most interesting review of the surgery of the Alexandrian School. He describes many instruments in detail, although he names fewer special instruments than some of the Greek writers as the Latin language lends itself less well to the formation of compound words than the Greek does. To take one example only, Celsus has practically one word for all varieties of forceps—vulsella, while the Greeks use many compounds like hair forceps (τριχο-λαβίς), flesh forceps (σαρκο-λάβος), tooth forceps (ὀδοντάγρα), stump forceps (ῥιζάγρα). Indeed, in the case of the two latter words Celsus falls back on Greek to express himself. Celsus was first published in 1478. Another edition is that of Targa, 1769. The editions before me are those of Daremberg, published at Leipzig in 1859, and Védrènes (Paris, 1876). The latter contains illustrations of a considerable number of specimens from Italian and French museums.

Rufus of Ephesus (98–117 A. D.) has left little to interest us for our particular purpose, as he merely mentions, without describing, a few instruments, all of which are already known to us from other sources. The best edition is that of Daremberg, Paris, 1879. A Latin translation of his works will be found in *Medicae Artis Principes* (Stephanus).

Aretaeus of Cappadocia has left us a work on Acute and Chronic Diseases. He has few references to instruments, but such as they are they are interesting, as he names some which are given by no other author. He has a tantalizing allusion to a work by himself on surgery which has not been preserved. There is a fine edition of the text, with an English translation by Adams of Banchory, in the Transactions of the Sydenham Society.

Galen (130–200 A. D.) was a most voluminous writer, much of whose work remains and teems with matter of interest to us. Much information about instruments is to be gained from even his purely anatomical writings. The most accessible edition is that of Kühn (20 vols., Leipzig, 1821), but it is slipshod in the text, and even more so in the translation, which is in Latin.

Oribasius (325 A. D.) wrote an encyclopaedia of medicine, which is called Συναγωγαὶ Ἰατρικαί—Collecta Medicinalia, in seventy books, only about one third of which remain. This is the most interesting of his works from our point of view, but he has left also a synopsis of the encyclopaedia called Σύνοψις, and a sort of first aid manual called Εὐπόριστα. I have used the edition of Daremberg and Bussemaker (1851–76).

Soranus of Ephesus has left us a most valuable treatise on obstetrics and gynaecology, which, though written only for midwives, contains many interesting references to instruments such as the speculum, uterine sound, cephalotribe, decapitator, and embryo hook. He lived in the reign of Trajan.. Some of the chapters, of which the Greek is lost, have been preserved to us by his abbreviator Moschion. I have used the edition of Rose published at Leipzig in 1882.

Moschion (fifth century) translated into Latin the gynae-cological and obstetrical part of the works of Soranus for the benefit of midwives who could not speak Greek. This version is now lost, but we have a translation of it into Greek, made after the fall of the Western Empire and the development of the Greek-speaking Empire at Constanti-nople in the sixth century. There is an Edition of this by Gesner (Basle, 1566). Finally, this Greek version of Moschion was translated back into barbarous Latin at some early date, Barbour thinks by some member of the Schola Salernitana. This was published at Venice by Aldus in the sixteenth century, and Rose has prefaced his edition of Soranus with it. This work of Moschion is only of interest to us from the fact that he preserves to us the substance of some chapters of which the original in Soranus is wanting.

Caelius Aurelianus Siccensis, an African of the fourth or fifth century, translated the works of Soranus, both those on gynaecology and those on general diseases, and he preserves some of Soranus which we would not otherwise possess ; but he writes in a barbarous Latin which, like the Latin of some other African writers on medical subjects, is calcu-lated to cause great pain to any one not familiar with this particular style.

Aetius lived in the first half of the sixth century, and compiled a voluminous treatise on medicine in sixteen books. He worked entirely with scissors and paste, but the result is the preservation to us of a large number of extracts from writers whose works would otherwise have entirely disappeared, and his work is of great value for the study of instruments. In 1534 an Aldine Edition of the first eight books was published, and, though a translation of the whole work was published by Cornarius in 1533–42 in

Latin, six of the last eight books were never published in the original Greek. This is unfortunate for us, as for our purpose the original is the only thing of any great value, Greek being, as I have already pointed out, a language richer in compounds than Latin is, and lending itself better to the coining of special names for special instruments. Not that the sixteenth-century translator is ever at a loss for a turn by which to express himself in Latin, but the turn, as often as not, is by periphrasis just at the very point when we would have liked a very exact equivalent for the Greek. The translation of the part of the work of which we have the Greek shows that we cannot entirely depend on some of these periphrases even where they appear definite, as in some cases an unwarrantable assumption is made about the form of an instrument. Thus λιθουλκῷ is translated 'forcipe ad id facta' because in Cornarius's time the instrument used for extracting stone from the bladder was a forceps, whereas it is doubtful whether there was in the Roman period anything more than a scoop, and, therefore, we are not entitled to translate λιθουλκός by anything more definite than 'stone extractor', its etymological equivalent. Although, therefore, I have examined the latter eight books of Aetius in the Latin translation, and although they contain some of the most interesting information to be found in the whole work, I have been very chary about laying stress on any deductions drawn from the Latin translation only. It may be noted that there are two ways of referring to the different books in Aetius, according to whether the Greek text or the translation of Cornarius is meant. Cornarius arranged his version in four tetrabibli of four books each, whereas the Greek text is simply numbered from i–viii. 'No vii.' of the Greek text is, therefore, called by Cornarius 'Tetr. ii. lib. iii.' The eleventh book was published by Daremberg in his edition of Rufus (1879), and the twelfth book was published by Costomeris at Paris in 1892.

Pliny the Younger. Plinius Secundus (Rose, Leipzig, 1875). The writings of Pliny contain little informa-

tion of any kind and are absolutely of no use for our
purpose.

Scribonius Largus (45 A. D.).   The edition I have examined
is named 'Scribonii Largi Compositiones' and is edited by
Helmreich, Leipzig, 1887.   The work of Scribonius Largus
is entirely pharmaceutical, but he gives many references to
appliances by which medicaments were prepared in the
surgery.

Marcellus Empiricus (300 A. D.) wrote a work on pharmacy,
of large size but little value, and in a poor style.   There are
a few passages bearing on implements of minor surgery.
A good deal is copied from Largus.   Aldus published the
text by Cornarius at Venice in his collection of Medici
Antiqui (1547), republished by Stephanus (*Medicae Artis
Principes*), 1567.   The edition I have used is that of Helmreich (Leipzig, 1889).

Theodorus Priscianus, alias Octavius Horatianus, lived in
the fourth century and has left a work, in three books, called
Euporiston.   It is a compilation in African Latin of extracts
from Galen, Oribasius, &c.   The style of the Latin is so
barbarous that it really must be seen to be believed.   There
is a little information to be gathered about minor instruments.   The edition I have used is that of Rose, Leipzig,
1894.   To this edition are tacked on the medical remains
of Vindicianus Afer, mere fragments without anything to
interest us.

The works of Alexander Trallianus (526–605 A. D.) contain
practically no surgery at all, although I have managed to
extract a few references of minor interest.

The last of the eminent Greek writers is Paulus Aegineta,
a writer who probably lived in the sixth and seventh
centuries.   This is getting rather late in the day, it is true,
but to omit the works of Paulus, or Paul, as he is affection-
ately called by his admirers, would be to omit some of the
most valuable knowledge of ancient medicine we possess.
Paul, like most of his time, was a compiler, but he was
a skilful one, and while he entirely depends on Galen,

Archigenes, Soranus, &c. for his information, he has gathered up the best of the medical knowledge of his time in a little encyclopaedia whose artistic completeness and orderly arrangement are not surpassed by any work of a corresponding nature at the present day. The work is divided into seven books, the sixth of which deals with surgery and teems with information about instruments. Aldus published the entire Greek text at Venice in 1527. A fine English translation, with a most valuable commentary, was published by Adams of Banchory for the Sydenham Society in 1846. No one who reads it can wonder that Adams had a worldwide reputation for his knowledge of medical history. The important sixth book was published along with a translation in French by Briau at Paris in 1855.

I have obtained a description of two very important instruments from the works of Hero of Alexandria (285–222 B.C., ed. 1575). There are a few interesting references to instruments in the works of the early Christian fathers. Tertullian is the only one of these I can claim to have systematically searched, but in one of his sermons he refers to no less than four surgical instruments, one of which is not described by any other author.

It were a work of supererogation to recount the names of the other Greek and Roman writers whose works I have run through in a profitless search for references to instruments. Some of these, such as Dioscorides, are of great importance in themselves though valueless for our purpose. Others, such as many of the minor Greek writers contained in the collection by Ideler entitled *Physici et Medici Graeci Minores* (Berlin, 1841), and the minor Latin writers contained in the collection of *Medici Antiqui Omnes* (Aldus, 1547), are of little value of any kind.

Before the capture of Alexandria by Omar in 651, many Greek medical writings had been translated into Syrian. At a later date such of these as had escaped destruction were turned into Arabic by the scholars of Bagdad (Honain and his School), in the ninth century. These, introduced into Spain in the Middle Ages by the Moors, were again translated into Latin and supplied for many a day the greater part of the medical knowledge of Europe, until the study of the few Greek texts which had escaped destruction showed the true origin of Arabian medicine. It will thus be seen that there is some information, in fact a great deal, to be had from the study of the works of the Arabs, but the barbarous style of the Latin and the roundabout way in which the works have been preserved, having passed through translations of three different languages, preclude any very exact deductions being drawn from them. Some of these works are profusely illustrated with figures of instruments, but I have been careful not to fall back on any of the Arabs except to support deductions drawn from more direct sources.

The chief Arab writers of interest to us are :—Serapion (800), Rhases (882), and Ali Abbas (after 950), all of Honain's School at Bagdad. The huge work of Avicenna (born 980), *The Canon*, was much used by the Arabs. It was published at Cordova, which became the Bagdad of the West after the Arabs crossed to Spain in 811.

The work of Albucasis (ob. 1106) was also published at Cordova, and contains much surgical information and has many illustrations of surgical instruments, but these must be used with due caution. I have used the edition published at Strasburg in 1532.

A word must be said of the later writers such as Paré (1509–90), Scultetus (1650), and Heister (1739). The works of these are profusely illustrated with instruments, some of which can plainly be seen to tally exactly with the descriptions of the classical authors. In other cases, although the names given to the instruments are those of classical times, it is, to say the least, doubtful whether they are of the same form as the ancient instruments whose names they bear. That was an age of great activity in the manufacture of new forms of surgical instruments, and we must accept with caution illustrations professing to indicate ancient forms of instruments. At the same time it is very interesting to note the large number of primitive arrangements which remained in use till nearly 1800. The enema syringe figured by Heister is exactly the same as we find described in the Hippocratic works—the bladder of an animal affixed to a tube—and many practitioners alive at the present day have seen the same simple arrangement in actual use.

CHAPTER II

MATERIAL, EXECUTION, AND ORNAMENTATION

Steel and Iron.

THE surgical instruments we meet with are, as a rule, of bronze. Not that the Greeks and Romans did not make many of their instruments of iron and steel, but the iron has mainly perished while more of the bronze has persisted. Long before the date of the earliest medical writings, Greece had passed into the iron age. The Homeric poems picture a civilization in the state of transition from a bronze to an iron period, and weapons such as sword, axe, and spear, are frequently described as made of iron. In the *Iliad* we even read of implements of agriculture made of iron, but it is 'hard to work' (πολύκμητος, *Iliad* vi. 48, *Od.* xxi. 10). However, by the time that Hippocrates wrote, it was in common use, and, if we had only the evidence of the Hippocratic writings to go by, we could see that it was in common use in the time of Hippocrates. Certain instruments, such as the cautery, are always spoken of as made of iron, in fact, the term for cautery is, as a rule, 'the iron,' and σίδηρος ὁ ὀξύς is a general term for 'the knife'. The smelting of iron is even used as a simile by Hippocrates:

'In the same way iron comes from stones and earth burnt together. In the first exposure to the fire stones and earth mix together with scoria, but at the second and third burning the scoria separate themselves from the iron, and this phenomenon meets the eye, that the iron remains in the fire fallen apart from the scoria, and becomes solid and compact' (ii. 371).

Again, he uses as a simile a speculative theory as to the way in which heating iron softens it and dipping it in water hardens it. He believes that this comes about by the fire depriving the iron of its nourishing substance, while the addition of water restores it.

Σιδήρου ὄργανα τέχνης· τὸν σίδηρον περιτήκουσι, πνεύματι ἀναγκά-
ζοντες τὸ πῦρ, τὴν ὑπάρχουσαν τροφὴν ἀφαιρέοντες, ἀραιὸν δὲ
ποιήσαντες, παίουσι καὶ συνελαύνουσιν. ὕδατος δὲ ἄλλου τροφῇ
ἰσχυρὸν γίνεται (ii. 641).

'The instruments of ironworking soften iron by driving
the fire with wind and taking away the supporting substance, and when they have rarefied it they strike and beat
it. By the nourishment of water it is again strengthened.'

This is the earliest reference to tempering steel by the
Greeks with which I am acquainted. It is a curious commentary on the relative destruction of iron instruments
compared with those of bronze, that cauteries, which are
always described as made of iron and which must have
existed in enormous numbers, are among the rarest surgical
instruments found. We have a few cauteries of iron, however, and some knives and knife-blades and other instruments remain. Pots for ointments of certain kinds were
made of iron, and we have actually two of these which
had been the property of a Roman oculist whose full
name is known. I have entered into this discussion because
there seems to be a general tendency to underestimate the
extent to which iron was employed by the Greeks and
Romans. The quantity of scoria left by the primitive
founders should alone be sufficient to teach us to how great
an extent iron was in use. Wherever there was good iron
in any of the Roman provinces, veritable mountains of scoria
are found. The heaps of scoria left in the Forest of Dean
by the Roman founders contained such a large percentage
of iron still remaining that they were smelted over again
in later times, and to do this occupied over twenty furnaces
for a couple of centuries. Tolouse calculated that similar
heaps in Gaul contained over 120,000 tons of scoria. If,
however, we tend to underestimate the extent to which
iron was in use among the Greeks and Romans, still more,
I believe, do we tend to underrate the quantity and the
quality of the steel available in those times. This comes
about from the fact that in our day we require such enormous quantities of iron and steel that we have to employ iron

ores of a very low quality. The greater part of the so-called
steel of which battleships are made is got from a ferruginous
mud with only 30 per cent. of iron, less than there was left
in the scoria after the Roman founder had done with it. To
the impurities already existing in this we add others,
because the coal we use contains sulphur. It is getting
rid of these impurities that makes the production of steel
such a roundabout process with us. We forget that, with
primitive methods but fine ores and a fuel devoid of sulphur, the production of steel of fine quality is as easy
a process as the manufacture of iron, in fact the only
difference between the method of procuring iron and
steel under these circumstances is the length of time
the process is allowed to go on. The ancient founders used
the finest ores, often containing 75 per cent. of iron, and,
working with charcoal fuel, which was nearly pure carbon,
they could produce steel as easily as iron. The difference between steel and iron is that steel contains carbon,
and, by allowing the ore to remain longer in contact with
the charcoal, steel is formed, so that a founder setting
out to make iron with a pure ore and a pure fuel like
charcoal, may, if he is not careful, turn out steel of fine
quality. This primitive method of making steel is still in
vogue in India, Burma, Borneo, China, &c., and very fine
qualities of steel are produced. The majority of the tools
found in the earliest Greek colonies on the Nile—Naukratis
and Daphnae—are of steel or iron, although those of the
Egyptians among whom they were living (circa 600 B. C.)
were of bronze. The classical medical writings themselves
are sufficient evidence of the quality of the steel available
in those times. Galen (ii. 683) says that the best quality
of steel (which came from Norica) yielded a knife which
neither blunted easily nor bent or chipped.

Ἐκ σιδήρου δὲ ἔστω τοῦτο τοῦ καλλίστου, οἷόν περ τὸ Νωρικόν
ἐστιν, ἵνα μήτ᾽ ἀμβλύνηται ταχέως, μήτ᾽ ἀνακάμπτηται ἢ θραύηται.

This shows that the Greek surgeon appreciated good steel,
and what I have said will show that there was plenty of it

to be had. Yet modern writers almost invariably speak of or describe even the cutting instruments of the ancients as made of iron. Greek and Latin have each only one word to indicate both steel and iron, but that is because, as I have shown, they prepared both in the same way. The ancient Hindoo Vedas say that cutting instruments were to be made of steel, well polished and sufficiently keen to divide a hair. For sharpening, a stone was to be used, and they were to be kept clean and wrapt in flannel and laid by in a box of sandalwood. Albucasis in mentioning steel always specifies Indian steel. Many of the Roman shears of steel retain their spring perfectly. As an illustration of the keenness of edge which can be put by simple methods upon steel of primitive manufacture, take the following account of the operations of an African barber of the Hausa tribe, as reported in an account by Professor R. W. Reid, Aberdeen, of a Hausa barber-doctor's outfit presented to the Anthropological Museum of the University by Sir William MacGregor, Governor of Lagos. The description of the outfit is quoted from Sir William MacGregor, who says:

'The knife, made by an African bush blacksmith, he uses for shaving. He employs no soap to soften the skin or roughen the hair, only a little water. He sharpens his razor on a black leather strap, turning the knife on the back so deftly that the eye cannot follow the movement; the few last touches he gives to it by turning it with splendid dexterity on the front of the left arm, where the skin is worn and bare by this manipulation. He shaves the whole face, except the nose. He leaves a fine line of eyebrow. The hair is cut short. The outline of the hairy part of the scalp in front is very clearly demarcated by shaving back about a half to an inch and a half. Then he turns the front edge by a marvellous stroke. He holds the knife horizontally, and, with a downward stroke cuts off all the projecting ends of the hair round the forehead. No European barber could do it without burying his razor in the skin. He never draws blood' (*Proc. Anat. and Anthrop. Soc. Univ. Abdn.*, 1900–2).

Bronze.

Although, as I have shown, iron and steel were largely used in the manufacture of instruments, fortunately for us bronze was the metal usually selected, for thus many instruments have withstood the lapse of time which would otherwise have been oxidized out of existence. Copper is much more easily got from ore than iron, and consequently it was the first to be used by man, and very early the advantage of combining it with tin to form bronze was found out. Bronze was used by the Egyptians 6,000 years ago, and the Phoenicians, who got it from them, passed it on to the whole of Europe. The quantity of tin in the bronze is very constantly about 7½ per cent.

The majority of the instruments which have been preserved to us are of bronze. Hippocrates (i. 58) says:

Χαλκώματι δὲ πλὴν τῶν ὀργάνων, μηδενὶ χρήσθω. καλλωπισμὸς γάρ τις εἶναί μοι δοκεῖ φορτικὸς σκεύεσι τοιουτέοισι χρῆσθαι.

'Use bronze only for instruments, for it seems laboured ornamentation to use vessels of it.'

We have, however, a good many specimens of vessels which prove, that physicians did not adhere to this advice. We know too that certain medicaments were intentionally stored in copper vessels. Scribonius says:

Deinde in patella aeris Cyprii super carbones posita infervescit, donec mellis habeat non nimium liquidi spissitudinem atque ita reponitur puxide aeris Cyprii (*Compositiones*, xxxvii).

Pure copper was occasionally used for instruments, and of these we have a few remaining, and vessels and instruments of it are frequently mentioned: 'Oportet autem moveri aquam ipsam rudicula vel spathomela aeris rubri' (Marcellus, *De Medicamentis*, xiv. 44). Coins were frequently made of brass (ὀρείχαλκος, *orichalcum*, *aurichalcum*), a mixture of copper, tin, and zinc, and in Pompeii there have been found two scalpel handles of brass composed of 25 per cent. of zinc and 75 per cent. of copper. The copper was got mainly from Cyprus and Spain. A small amount, however, came from Africa and Asia.

Tin.

Tin came mainly from Britain. We have no instruments of tin preserved to us, but they are frequently referred to. Hippocrates mentions, over and over again, uterine sounds of tin, and he also speaks of sounds and eyed probes for rectal work, which were made of tin so that they might be flexible. Vessels of tin for storing medicaments in are spoken of by Largus: 'Reponitur medicamentum fictili vel stagneo vase' (cclxviii). In the Museum at Chesters (Chollerford) there is a tin weight for medicines.

Lead.

Leaden sounds and tubes for intra-uterine medication are frequently mentioned in the Hippocratic writings, and Celsus and Paul refer to leaden tubes for insertion in the rectum and vagina to prevent cicatricial contractions and adhesions after operations on these parts. The therapists also mention medicament jars of lead. There is one in the Capitoline Museum from the temple of Aesculapius in the forum.

Gold.

There is in the Museum at Stockholm a forceps of gold, but it is more than probable that this is a toilet article. I have a spatula-probe which had been overlaid with gold, and I have met with several others similarly treated. Theodorus Priscianus recommends a cautery of gold for stopping haemorrhage from the throat (*Logicus*, xxii). Avenzoar speaks of a golden probe for applying salve to the eye and for separating adhesion of the eye to the lid. Avicenna lets out the pustules of small-pox with a golden probe. Albucasis recommends burning the roots of hairs in trichiasis with a probe of gold. Mesue recommends a heated scalpel of gold to excise the tonsil. Hippocrates binds the teeth together in fracture of the jaw with a gold wire (iii. 174); cf. Paul, VI. xcii. In one of his dialogues Lucian satirizes a medical man who sought to conceal his ignorance by a display of a fine library, bleeding-cups of silver, and scalpel handles inlaid with gold—the devices of quacks, Lucian says, who did not know how to use the instruments when necessity arose.

Silver.

There is a forceps of silver in the Athens Museum, and another in the Museum at Kiel. Both are, however, possibly toilet articles. Paul condemns bleeding-cups of silver, as he says they burn, so it is evident that Lucian had grounds for his statement. In the Musée de Cinquantenaire, Brussels, there is in the section of ancient surgery a bronze instrument case from Pompeii which contained a silver spoon and probe combined, a plain probe, and a grooved director, all in silver. I have frequently met with ligulae of silver and also of copper overlaid with silver, and styli, which we shall see were used as implements of minor surgery, were frequently made of silver. Medicament boxes of silver are mentioned by Marcellus. Hippocrates describes a uterine syringe with a tube of silver. Albucasis mentions silver catheters.

A mixture of gold and silver, which was called electrum, was much used for coinage, and I have met with one or two ligulae of this metal. It was found mixed naturally in the mountain districts of Tmolus and Sipylus in Lydia, and it was also artificially produced by alloying the two metals.

Horn.

Hippocrates (iii. 331) speaks of a pessary of horn inserted into the rectum. It would seem that the tube of various syringes was often made of horn, as both Greek and Latin writers speak of the 'horn' of the syringe.

Scribonius Largus (*Compositiones*, vii) says:

Per nares ergo purgatur caput his rebus infusis per cornu, quod rhinenchytes vocatur (cf. Galen, xi. 125).

Wood.

Galen speaks of sounds or directors of wood, and ointment spatulae of wood are very frequently mentioned in the therapeutic works, as are also boxes for storing ointments in.

Bone and Ivory.

Numbers of bone ligulae were found in a Roman hospital lately excavated at Baden.

In the Naples Museum there are two ointment spoons with carved bone handles. Needles such as Hippocrates and Celsus speak of for stitching bandages to fix them were very frequently made of bone and ivory. Knife handles of bone and ivory are common. A carved ivory medicament box with sliding lid will be fully described later. Scribonius Largus describes knives of bone and ivory for preparing plants for pharmaceutical purposes (*Compositiones*, lxxxiii). An ivory pestle was found with a surgeon's outfit in Cologne.

Stone.

Medicaments were prepared on stone slabs, and the great majority of oculists' seals were of stone.

Execution and Ornamentation.

The execution of the instruments is, as a rule, all that could be desired, and the weight and thickness are no more than is consistent with the requisite strength.

Hippocrates points out the necessity for this :—

Τἀδ' ὄργανα πάντα εὐήρη πρὸς τὴν χρείαν ὑπάρχειν δεῖ τῷδε μεγέθει, καὶ βάρει, καὶ λεπτότητι.

'All instruments ought to be well suited for the purpose in hand as regards their size, weight, and delicacy' (i. 58).

The ornamentation is simple and effective. In the round instruments like the probes it consists usually of raised circular ornamentation, with or without a secondary ornamentation on the raised ringing. In others there are longitudinal or spiral grooves running along the instrument. In some cases the bronze is decorated with an inlay of silver damascening. This is rare in the instruments from Pompeii, though there are two probes with a spiral inlay in the Naples Museum. The majority of the instruments treated in this way have been found in the western

provinces, and they are of later date than the Pompeian.
The handles of some scalpels belonging to the third century
are beautifully inlaid with silver.   Lucian, as I have
mentioned, speaks of scalpels inlaid with gold.   In the
Mainz Museum there is a medicament box on the lid of
which is inlaid a snake coiled round a tree, the tree and
the snake's body being outlined in copper and the snake's
head in silver.   So far no damascened instruments are
reported from Greece.   Damascening began in Europe
apparently in the first century, and reached its height in
the time of the Merovingian kings.

Examples of plated instruments are not uncommon.   I
have a spatula dissector thinly plated with gold, and I have
met with several ligulae plated with silver.   One of these
was so thickly plated that on cutting into it the silver,
which was deeply oxidized on the outside and was, therefore,
quite black, showed also a layer of metallic silver still bright
on section.

All the surgical instruments found in the provinces have
an *air de famille* which would lead one to suppose that they
had been manufactured in Italy, but this is not certain.
The ointment slabs, however, are rarely of the stone of the
country in which they are found.   On the other hand, the
orthographical faults on the oculists' seals would indicate
that they were cut in the provinces.   Wherever possible
two instruments are combined into one.   Thus very few of
the probes are simple instruments but carry a spatula,
a scoop or spoon, an eye, or a hook, at the opposite end.
Vulsella are more difficult to combine with other instruments, but here again we meet with combinations such as
vulsella at one end and scoop, raspatory, or probe, at the
other.   The typical scalpel handle carries at the end
opposite the blade a spatula for blunt dissection.   We have
needles at one end and probes, scalpel blades, &c., at the
other end of a handle.   This combination of two instruments
in one is still in use in our day.   We must notice the fact
that the majority of instruments we know were all of metal,

not folding into hollow handles of wood, bone, &c., as the instruments of a decade ago did, so that they were easily cleaned. In fact we shall see that where the scalpel and handle were not forged in one piece they were united by something very like our aseptic joint. Hippocrates insists on the importance of keeping everything in the surgery absolutely clean.

A few instruments bear the image of deities connected with medicine, or attributes of these. The figures of Aesculapius and his daughter Hygeia are found on medicament boxes, the former with the serpent entwining his staff, the latter feeding a serpent from a bowl. The serpent is sometimes found on a probe. A uterine dilator from Pompeii also carries it. A probe surmounted by a double serpent (caduceus form) was found in the Roman Hospital at Baden. Two scalpels in the Naples Museum carry on their ends the head of Minerva Medica. The quadrivalve speculum in the Naples Museum has each end of the crossbar tipped with a fine image of a ram's head. There is also a medicine shovel with the same symbol. Illustrations of these instruments will be found later.

Preservation.

Some of the instruments of silver retain their brightness as when they were made, but under certain circumstances a considerable amount of oxidation takes place, and then they have a thick black coating. Very few bronze articles are found to have retained their colour. In volcanic districts the various sulphur compounds formed give rise to a beautiful patina of varying shades of green and blue, sometimes so evenly distributed as to resemble enamel. This, when fine, much enhances the value of the article.

Articles of iron are sometimes but little destroyed. It is surprising in how good condition the iron or steel may be. The bow of a shears is sometimes quite springy. In some cases a steel or iron article is often represented by a mass of oxide bearing some resemblance to the original. In others only a shapeless mass of oxide remains.

Finds of Instruments.

Finds of ancient surgical instruments, though not by any means common, are still sufficiently numerous for specimens to have found their way into most of our larger museums; and private collectors have here and there acquired considerable numbers. The most prolific source has been the excavations at Herculaneum and Pompeii, which have now been systematically pursued for nearly three hundred years, while the objects found have been deposited in the National Museum at Naples. In 1818 a physician's house with a large number of surgical instruments was discovered in the Strada del Consulare of Pompeii, and two chemists' shops have also been found with instruments in them. Besides these there is a large number of instruments from other finds in the two buried cities.

The custom of burying personal effects along with the ashes of a deceased person, which prevailed among the Romans from the second to the fourth century, has preserved to us a number of interesting finds. In 1880 M. Tolouse, a civil engineer in Paris, in executing some alterations in the neighbourhood of the Avenue Choisy, discovered the grave of a surgeon, containing a bronze pot full of surgical instruments. Among these were numerous forceps and vulsella, ointment tubes, bleeding cup, scalpel handles for blades of steel, probes, and spatulae. Sixty-six coins of the reigns of Tetricus I and II showed that the grave belonged to the end of the second or the beginning of the third century. The find was reported by M. Tolouse in a volume entitled *Mes fouilles dans le sol du vieux Paris* (Paris, 1888). In 1892 the find was fully described by Professor Deneffe of Ghent, in the *Revue Archéologique*, under the title ' Notice descriptive sur une trousse de médecin au IIIme siècle ', and reprinted, with photogravures, in 1893 in a monograph *Étude sur la trousse d'un chirurgien Gallo-Romain du IIIme siècle* (Antwerp, 1893). It is convenient to refer to this find as that of the ' Surgeon of

Paris '.   Another grave containing surgical instruments was found at Wancennes in the canton of Beauraing, Namur, in a cemetery of the first or second century.   The instruments are now in the Archaeological Museum at Namur (Deneffe, op. cit., p. 35).

In 1854 there were discovered at Rheims the remnants of a wooden chest containing two little iron jars for ointments, several scalpel handles, a small drill, eight handles for needles, five hooks (two blunt and three sharp), two balances, various probes and spatulae, seven forceps, medicament box, a mortar, and a seal showing that the instruments had belonged to an oculist named Gaius Firmius Severus. The instruments are all of the most beautiful pattern and finish, several being finely inlaid with silver.   Some coins of the reigns of Antoninus Pius and Marcus Aurelius showed that the interment belonged to the end of the third century.

These instruments, &c., are now in the Museum of St-Germain-en-Laye.   The majority of these will be found described and figured later.

Find of Sextus Polleius Sollemnis, oculist of Fonviel, Saint-Privat-d'Allier.   In levelling a heap of earth which had fallen from a cliff above as the result of a landslide, there were found at Fonviel in 1864 a number of bronze surgical instruments.   The place where they were found is at the intersection of two old Roman roads, and the instruments had been buried in the grave of a Roman surgeon high up above the valley on the edge of a cliff.   Eighteen coins of the reigns of Julia Augusta, Trajan, Hadrian, Commodus, Gordian, Philip, Valerian, and Gallus, showed that the interment had been made at the end of the third century.   The instruments found included three scalpel handles, fragments of two forceps, and an oculist's seal in stone showing that the grave was that of Sextus Polleius Sollemnis.   Many more instruments had probably been buried originally.   Those enumerated are now in the Museum of Le Puy-en-Velay.   An account of this find, with illustrations, is to be found in the *Annales de la Société d'Agriculture, Sciences, Arts et Commerce du Puy* (tome xxvi. 1864–5). It is also described, along with the find of Gaius Firmius Severus, in a monograph by Deneffe, under the title of *Les Oculistes Gallo-Romains au* iiime *siècle* (Antwerp, 1896).

One of the most prolific finds of late years has been the discovery of a Roman military hospital at Baden, the ancient Roman station of Aquae, or Vicus Aquensis. From time to time isolated discoveries of instruments had been made, including a catheter, a scalpel, and several varieties of probes, and in March, 1893, MM. Kellersberger and Meyer proceeded to excavate systematically the remains of some Roman buildings on their property. A large chamber 10·35 metres by 12·5, with walls 60 cm. thick, was discovered, and later others were discovered varying from 3 to 27 metres in length. There were in all fourteen rooms. Along the side of the building on which a Roman road ran, there were the remains of an imposing façade, running the whole length of the building. It had consisted of a portico with colonnades, the foundations of which were found at regular intervals. It is possible that some of the larger rooms had been subdivided into others by thin walls or partitions, for fragments of partitions of plaster with wood lathing were found.

A large number of objects—tiles, lamps, vases, pots, knives, spearheads, nails, glass, fibulae, beads, weavers' weights, three amphorae a metre high—were found near the surface. Then, at a depth of two metres, surgical instruments began to be found. These included probes to the number of 120, unguent spoons in bone and bronze, a fragment of a catheter 13 cm. long, bronze boxes for powder, needles, earscoops, unguentaria, spatulae, a fragment of an étui for instruments, and cauteries. Many coins of the reigns of Claudius, Nero, Domitian, Vespasian, and Hadrian were found, showing that the hospital had been in use between 100 and 200 A.D. The objects mentioned are still the private property of MM. Kellersberger and Meyer. In 1905, by the kindness of these gentlemen, I was allowed to make a complete examination of the collection.

A case containing a surgeon's outfit was found in the Luxemburgerstrasse, Cologne. It contained a phlebotome, a chisel, and some fragments of other instruments of steel, two forceps and two sharp hooks in bronze, and a small ivory pestle-like instrument. These are now in the Cologne Museum. This is a most interesting and important little find. The phlebotome is by far the best preserved and best authenticated example which we possess of this instrument. Probably the same may be said of the chisel as a purely surgical instrument.

CHAPTER III

KNIVES

THE surgical knife had, as a rule, the blade of steel and the handle of bronze. We find specimens all of steel or all of bronze but these are exceptional forms; and hence it happens that many more handles than blades have been preserved to us, as usually the blade has oxidized away leaving no trace of its shape. It will be well, therefore, to commence with the study of the handle.

The scalpel handle consists, as a rule, of a bar of bronze, which may be round, square, hexagonal, or trapezoidal in section. At one end there is a slot to receive the steel blade, varying in depth from 2 cm. in the larger, to 1 cm. in the smaller, instruments. The other end of the handle carried a leaf-shaped spatula to act as a blunt dissector. A groove is often formed near the end of the handle, or the end is raised into a cylindrical roll on each side, and this roll again is sometimes perforated with a hole.

It is generally believed that the blades were fixed in the handle by a binding thread or wire, and that the rolls and perforations were to give security to the mounting used. This detachable arrangement would allow of removal for cleaning, and also permit one handle to be used with several varieties of blade. A consideration of the slots in a large number of handles leads me to believe, however, that this was, to say the least, not the usual arrangement. The proportion of the depth of the slot to the size of the blade to be supported is in most cases not large enough to allow of a temporary mounting to fix the blade firmly, and I believe that most blades were either luted or brazed in permanently.

These processes were well known to the ancients, and in fact we have them in evidence in other surgical instruments. Those bleeding-cups from Pompeii which carry rings on their summits have the top part brazed or soldered on. Galen (ii. 717) alludes to the blowpipe which goldsmiths used, and Paulus Aegineta has a chapter on the fluxes used by these artists. We frequently meet with ornaments fixed on boxes by means of solder.

On the other hand, the slot in some handles expands at its termination into a wider portion which would carry a cylindrical expansion on the other end of the blade. This form of blade could not be pulled outwards, and might well be fixed with a temporary mounting.

Different varieties of handles are shown in Plates I–III. Some are beautifully damascened with silver. These are mostly of the third century, but Sambon reports some damascened handles of the first century. A rare form is seen in a specimen in the Museum at Le Puy-en-Velay, where the handle is round and decorated with a spiral band of silver inlaid round it. It is from the find of the oculist Sollemnis (Pl. II, fig. 6).

A few variations from the characteristic combination of handle and spatula-shaped dissector occur. Thus we have a handle ending in a conical point (Pl. II, fig. 7), which Deneffe regards as a drill for perforating the nasal septum in cases of fistula lachrymalis. Archigenes describes this operation, and the handle was found in the grave of the oculist Severus. Along with it were found two other handles, which, instead of a spatula, had carried a steel needle (Pl. II, figs. 1, 2). The needles have disappeared of course, but there are the holes to receive them. In other cases the handle was round, and either quite plain or ornamented with raised rings. Some of these ended in a small round knob (Pl. V, fig. 2). Others carry the head of Minerva Medica like the spoon in Pl. XX, fig. 5. There are three of these handles in the Naples Museum. Rufus of Ephesus describes a lithotomy knife which had a scoop at the end of the handle with which to extract the stone. An example of this is seen in the box of scalpels from Athens (Pl. IV).

The Blade.

For the study of the different varieties of blade we have at our disposal first of all the specimens that have actually survived. Of these the largest number are to be seen in the Naples Museum, but a considerable number are to be found scattered over various museums. An *ex voto* tablet found on the site of the temple of Aesculapius on the Acropolis at Athens shows a box of scalpels, among which are some interesting forms (Pl. IV). The scalpels, it will be noted, are arranged head and tail alternately. A few varieties are actually described in detail in the classical authors, and, by piecing together other references to particular instruments and drawing inferences from the various uses to which we find them put, we are able to describe a surprisingly large number of forms. The sixteenth-century writers, such as Paré, and seventeenth-century writers, such as Scultetus, illustrate with great confidence many of the cutting instruments mentioned by ancient writers, but it is easy to show that in several instances they are wrong, and, therefore, I have drawn on them as little as possible.

As a basis of classification we may select the following points about the blade. The form may be straight or curved. There may be only one cutting edge or there may be two, and the point may be sharp or blunt. We shall examine combinations of these in the following order :

I. Blade straight—

 (A) Cutting on one side only (*a*) sharp-pointed,
  (*b*) blunt-pointed.

 (B) Cutting on two edges (*a*) sharp-pointed, (*b*) blunt-pointed.

II. Blade curved—

 (A) Cutting on one edge (*a*) sharp-pointed, (*b*) blunt-pointed.

 (B) Cutting on two edges, sharp-pointed.

I. A (a) *Straight blade cutting on one edge, sharp-pointed.*

1. Ordinary scalpel.
2. Scalpel with tip turned back.
3. Bellied scalpel.
4. Scolopomachaerion.

Ordinary Scalpel.

The ordinary scalpel had apparently a straight, sharp-pointed blade. The word which Galen, Aetius, and Paulus Aegineta use to denote scalpel is σμίλη. Latin authors use *scalpellus*, the diminutive of *scalper*. From the etymology of these terms we can learn nothing as to the shape of the blade; they are merely general terms denoting a cutting blade of any kind—chisel, graving tool, knife, &c. The word Hippocrates uses, μάχαιρα or μαχαίριον, has a more definite meaning. It is from μάχαιρα, the old Lacedaemonian sword, a broad blade cutting on one edge, sharp-pointed, and straight or with the tip turned slightly backwards. Thus, even in Hippocratic times the scalpel was apparently much of the same shape as it is now. Good examples of the ordinary scalpel may be seen in Pl. V, figs. 1 and 2 from the British Museum. They are all of steel. A variety with the point turned back at the tip is seen in one of the scalpels in the scalpel box from the Acropolis (Pl. IV).

A more bellied form is seen in Pl. V, fig. 5, which is from the Naples Museum, and is all of bronze, handle and blade. At the Scientific Congress held at Naples in 1845 Vulpes showed this specimen, and described it as the lithotomy knife invented by Meges and mentioned by Celsus (VII. xxvi).

Later I shall discuss in detail the instrument of Meges, but I believe the instrument shown by Vulpes is only an ordinary scalpel with a somewhat bellied shape.

Hippocrates refers to a bellied scalpel in a well-known passage on empyema (ii. 258):

Ὅκως σοι ἡ ἔξοδος τοῦ πύους εὐρὺς ᾖ τάμνειν δεῖ μεταξὺ τῶν πλευρῶν στηθοειδεῖ μαχαιρίδι τὸ πρῶτον δέρμα.

'Incise the outer integument between the ribs with a bellied scalpel.'

Στηθοειδής means rounded like the breast of a woman. Galen translates it in his lexicon τῷ σμιλίῳ ἰατρικῷ γαστρώδεῖ, 'the bellied surgical knife.' It is quite a serviceable instrument for several kinds of work, and it seems to have been a common form. Three out of the six scalpels depicted in the votive tablet from the Acropolis are of this form, and there are now in the Naples Museum four others of the same shape as the one described by Vulpes. These have blades of steel and handles of bronze. The figures of three of these (Pl. V, figs. 3–6), show the gradual evolution from a common scalpel into the bellied form. I have seen a scalpel with a blade similar to Pl. V, fig. 3 in use in Scotland for castrating piglings and calves.

Scarificator for wet cupping.

Paul (VI. xli) says that some have conceived for the purpose of scarifying before wet cupping an instrument compounded of three blades joined together in such a way that at one stroke three scarifications are made :

Τινὲς οὖν ἐπενόησαν ὄργανον πρὸς τοῦτο, τρία σμιλία ἴσα ζεύξαντες ὁμοῦ, ὅπως τῇ μιᾷ ἐπιβολῇ τρεῖς γίνοιντο διαιρέσεις.

Paul says he prefers a single scalpel.

What the precise shape of scalpel used was we cannot say, but it would most likely be one of the bellied forms. Hippocrates, in his treatise *De Medico*, says that the lancets used in wet cupping should be rounded and not too narrow at the tip (καμπύλοις ἐξ ἄκρου μὴ λίην στενοῖς). Even if καμπύλος meant curved and not bellied it would not be certain that it was meant to cut on the convex side of the blade. The words of Hippocrates imply at any rate a blade with a rounded, not sharp point (i. 62).

Straight sharp-pointed bistoury.

Greek, σκολοπομαχαίριον, σκολόπιον ; Latin, *scalpellus*. The etymology of the term σκολοπομαχαίριον as applied to a cutting instrument sufficiently indicates its shape. It takes its name from its similarity to the beak of a snipe, which is long and slender[1]. We find it used by Galen (xi. 1011) for dissecting out warts, excising caruncles from the inner canthus, puncturing the foetal cranium in obstructed labour, &c.

In Aetius (IV. iv. 23) and Paulus Aegineta (VI. lxxiv) it is used for opening not only the foetal cranium but also the thorax and abdomen of the foetus in transverse presentations. Paul refers to it for opening the thorax in empyema (VI. xliv) and the abdomen in ascites (VI. l). In both cases the outer integument was incised with a scalpel and the deeper layer punctured with the bistoury. In opening the abdomen for ascites, by sliding the outer skin upwards before the peritoneal cut was made, a valvular opening was secured. Although many other interesting applications of this instrument are to be found, these instances will suffice to show that the uses to which the instrument was put agree with the supposition that it was of the shape indicated by the etymology of its name. A variant form of the same name is σκολόπιον which also occurs pretty often.

A large variety of this instrument is mentioned by Galen as devised by him for the dissection of the spinal cord. He says he uses a knife of the same shape as the scolopomachaerion, but larger and stouter and made of the best Norican steel, so as to neither blunt, bend, nor break easily (ii. 682).

I. A (b) *Straight blade cutting on one side, blunt-pointed.*

(α) Novacula or razor (Greek ξυρόν, diminutive ξύριον).

(β) Blunt-pointed bistoury.

(γ) Ring knife for dismembering foetus.

Razor.

Shaving and cutting the hair were looked upon as important means of treatment in several diseases. Ori-

---

[1] So says Briau (*Paul D'Egine*, p. 97), but it seems more likely to be derived from σκόλοψ 'a spike'.

basius (*Med. Coll.* xxv) has a chapter on this entitled περὶ κουρᾶς καὶ ξυρήσεως. 'These things,' he says, 'have been introduced into medicine as a means of evacuation and as remedies in chronic diseases.'

Celsus makes frequent mention of shaving as a means of treatment. Of alopecia he says :

Sed nihil melius est quam novacula quotidie radere—quia, cum paulatim summa pellicula excisa est, adaperiuntur pilorum radiculae. Neque ante oportet desistere quam frequentem pilum nasci apparuerit (VI. iv).

A large scalpel of this form from the Naples Museum is shown in Pl. VI, fig. 1. The handle is of the usual shape and is made of bronze. The blade is of steel. It measures 15 cm. all over, the blade being 2 cm. broad at the heel. The cutting border slopes backward to the back of the blade, which is in a straight line with the border of the handle. At the point the blade is 1·5 cm. broad. It may be noted that this instrument had much the same shape as the *culter*, but *culter* is not a term applied by any Latin author to a surgical instrument, nor is *cultellus*, although the sixteenth-century translators of Aetius and Paulus Aegineta very frequently use the latter term. Scultetus figures a scalpel of this form and sums up its uses well :

La fig. est un rasoir ou scalpel droit ne tranchant que d'un coste et de l'autre mousse, dont les chirurgiens se servent lorsqu'il ne faut avoir aucun égard aux parties sujettes, scavoir lorsqu'il s'agit de faire des incisions au cuir de la teste jusqu'au crane, &c.

Another specimen also of this class, but with the blade so long in proportion to its width as to deserve the name of a blunt-pointed bistoury was excavated in a third-century graveyard at Stree, and is now in the Charleroi Museum. It is 14 cm. long by 1 cm. broad at the heel, widening gradually towards the point where it is 2 mm. broader than at the heel. The end of the blade is square (Pl. VI, fig. 2). An example of the domestic *culter* or *cultellus* is shown in Pl. VII, fig. 4. It is from a Roman camp at Sandy in Bedfordshire.

In the curious pseudo-Hippocratic treatise (i. 463) a knife to fix on the thumb and dismember a foetus in utero is mentioned :

Ἔχειν δὲ χρὴ πρὸς τὰ τοιαῦτα καὶ ὄνυχα ἐπὶ τῷ δακτύλῳ τῷ μεγάλῳ. καὶ διελόντα ἐξενεγκεῖν τὰς χεῖρας κτλ.

'If, however, the foetus be dead and remain, and cannot either spontaneously or with the aid of drugs come away in the natural manner, having liberally anointed the hand with cerate and inserted it in the uterus endeavour to separate the shoulders from the neck with the thumb. It is necessary to have for this a 'claw' upon the thumb and, the amputation having been performed, to extract the arms and, again inserting the hand, to open the abdomen and, having done so to remove the intestines, &c.'

An instrument answering to this description is still in use by veterinary surgeons (Pl. VII, fig. 1), but the forefinger, and not the thumb, is used. A scalpel blade is mounted on a ring and the forefinger is passed through the ring. Foals and calves are in this way easily dismembered in exactly the same way as is described by Hippocrates. The name of the instrument of Hippocrates would rather indicate that its blade was curved, but as the modern instrument has a probe point I have included it in this class. It is called by Tertullian the 'ring knife'—'cum annulo cultrato (var. lect. anulocultro) quo intus membra caeduntur anxio arbitrio' (*De Anima*, 26).

I. B (*a*) *Straight blade cutting on two edges, sharp-pointed.*

(1) Galen's 'long' dissecting knife.

(2) Phlebotome.

(3) Lithotome.

(4) Polypus knife.

Galen's knife for opening the vertebral canal.

In his description of the dissection of the spine Galen describes a large straight two-edged knife (ii. 682) :

Καθίημι τὸ πρόμηκες μαχαίριον, οὕτω γὰρ αὐτὸ καλῶ δύο πλευρὰς ὀξείας ἔχον ἐπὶ τοῦ πέρατος εἰς μίαν κορυφὴν ἀνηκούσας.

'I push in the 'long scalpel', for thus I describe the one with two cutting edges meeting in one at the tip.'

What Galen means by πρόμηκες when applied to an instrument he has himself explained in a note on the chapter by Hippocrates on the treatment of dislocation of the shoulder. He applies it to instruments long in proportion to their breadth (see p. 118). The knife referred to here is a large strong instrument, for it is intended for cutting through the lateral processes of the vertebrae.

Phlebotome.

Greek, φλεβοτόμον, τὸ (sc. σμιλίον), also φλεβοτόμος, ὁ (Galen). ὀξυβελές (sc. ὄργανον); Latin, phlebotomum (late), scalpellus.

Although venesection is one of the most frequently mentioned operations, and although the phlebotome is one of the most frequently named instruments, we have no passage giving even the most meagre description of this instrument. It is assumed that its appearance would be familiar to every one, since phlebotomy was so common. Celsus tells us that every one old and young was bled.

Sanguinem, incisa vena, mitti, novum non est, sed nullum paene morbum esse in quo non mittatur novum est (II. x).

The operation continued just as frequent all through the Roman period, and the writings on venesection are very voluminous. Galen has three treatises on the subject. The operation was performed in exactly the same way as at the present day, and the lancet was apparently the same as that figured in modern instrument catalogues, viz. sharp-pointed, double-edged, and straight. A consideration of all the various operations to which the phlebotome was put bears this out. The following passage from Hippocrates shows that there were various sizes of the phlebotome :

Τοῖς γε μαχαιρίοις ὀξέσι δεῖ χρῆσθαι καὶ πλάτεσι, οὐκ ἐπὶ πάντων ὁμοίως παραγγέλλομεν, κτλ. (i. 60).

' We do not recommend that the lancets narrow and broad should be used indiscriminately in all cases, for there are certain parts of the body which have a swift current of blood which it is not easy to stop. Such are varices and certain other veins. Therefore, it is necessary in these to make narrow openings, for otherwise it is not possible to stop the flow. Yet it is sometimes necessary to let blood from them. But in places not dangerous, and about which the blood is not thin, we use the lancets broader (πλατυτέροις χρῆσθαι τοῖς μαχαιρίοις), for thus and not otherwise will the blood flow.'

The phlebotome appears to have been a convenient instrument for all sorts of operations besides phlebotomy, especially for the opening of abscesses and the puncture of cavities containing fluid, and for fine dissecting work. Paulus Aegineta mentions its application for the excision of fistula lachrymalis (VI. xxii), the removal of warts (VI. lxxxvii), slitting the prepuce in phimosis (VI. lv), incising the tunica vaginalis in excision of hydrocele sac (VI. lxii), opening abscesses (VI. xxvii), dissection of sebaceous cysts (VI. xiv). Galen (xiv. 787) mentions its use in dissecting open an imperforate vagina. Celsus has no special word for phlebotome. He always refers to it by the general term scalpellus. Theodorus Priscianus, whose Latin takes curious forms, gives us a transliteration of the Greek term :

Convenit interea prae omnibus etiam his flebotomum adhibere, convenit etiam eos ventris purgatione iuvari (*Euporiston*, xxi. 66).

Hippocrates in the famous passage on the surgical treatment of empyema (ii. 258) says :

' Incise the skin between the ribs with a bellied scalpel, then let a phlebotome (ὀξυβελεῖ) which has been wound round with a rag, leaving the breadth of the thumb nail at the point, be pushed in.'

'Οξυβελής literally means sharp-pointed. The term occurs in the *Iliad*, e. g. applied to an arrow (iv. 126), but Galen in his Lexicon expressly states that Hippocrates by it means the phlebotome. In his treatment of empyema Paulus Aegineta uses not the phlebotome but a sharp curved bistoury; however, in opening the abdomen for ascites it is the phlebotome he recommends:

' We take a curved bistoury or a phlebotome and, having with the point of the instrument dissected the skin that lies over the peritoneum, we divide the peritoneum a little higher up than the first incision, and insert a tube of bronze.'

All these various applications of the phlebotome are consistent with the supposition that the phlebotome was the same as that figured in the catalogues of the present day. Heister says:

Spectant huc primo loco ea quae Tab. 1 sub litt. A & B (Pl. VII, figs. 6, 7) exhibentur, *scalpellum* nempe minus et maius; vulgus *lancettas* eadem nominant. Serviunt eadem, praesertim minora, venis incidendis, quare phlebotoma Graecis vocantur; sed et abscessibus aperiendis, imprimis maiora; ideoque Gallis etiam *lancettes a l'absces* appellari consueverunt.

A bronze blade of this shape is shown in Pl. VII, fig. 3. It was found near Rome.

The identity in shape of the abscess knife and the phlebotome holds good to-day. The best example of the phlebotome is in the Cologne Museum. It was found in the Luxemburgerstrasse along with the other contents of a surgeon's case. It is all of steel, with a square handle and blade of myrtle leaf shape (Pl. VII, fig. 2). There is in the Naples Museum an instrument which is of this shape, and Vulpes (Tav. VI, fig. 1) has described it as a lancet for bleeding. The instrument, however, is formed of a blade of silver set in a handle of bronze, so that it can scarcely be regarded as a cutting instrument (see Pl. XIX, fig. 2). I look upon it as an unguent spatula. There is, however, an instrument of bronze of phlebotome shape in the Naples Museum. It was found in the house of the physician in the Strada del Consulare of Pompeii, and it was described by Vulpes as an instrument for removing the eschar formed by a cautery, as it was found lying alongside a small trident-shaped cautery. It is doubtful whether the eschar formed by a cautery was removed at all, and it is still more doubtful whether Vulpes is justified in postulating a special instrument for doing so, and as this instrument is of phlebotome shape it is more likely to have been a phlebotome than anything else. It is of bronze, 8 cm. long and 9 mm. in the broadest part of the blade. The handle is neatly decorated with raised ring ornamentation.

The following account of the discovery of a phlebotome in excavating some graves along the line of the old Watling Street Road, in the neighbourhood of Wroxeter, is given by C. Roach Smith in the *Gentleman's Magazine* (1862, pt. ii. p. 677):

'Several sepulchral interments have been met with of a character similar to those usually found in Roman cemeteries. In some of them objects of particular interest were found, with urns and other earthen vessels; as, for instance, the fragments of a circular mirror in the bright, shining, mixed metal commonly known as 'speculum' metal; and what appears to be a surgeon's lancet, contrived in a very ingenious manner. The point for penetrating the flesh is of steel, not unlike that in use at the present day. It is surmounted by a guard to hinder it from cutting too deeply, and above this is a handle, which is bow-shaped, and of bronze.'

J. Corbet Anderson, in *The Roman City at Wroxeter*, p. 92, says it was embedded in the remains of a case in which it had been carried, and he gives an illustration of it (Pl. VII, fig. 5). A similar object is classified as a surgical instrument in the Louvre, but both these articles are I believe detached mirror handles. The passage quoted from Hippocrates shows that the ordinary phlebotome was not guarded in this way. A phlebotome of the principle of the fleam is figured by Albucasis and the method of using it in dividing the frontal vein by striking it with a comb is described. There is also a similar instrument in the Naples Museum, from Pompeii, which is classed as a veterinary instrument (Pl. VIII, fig. 3). It is probable, however, that such an instrument was used by Roman physicians, as the offices of surgeon and veterinarian were often held by the same individual in

Roman times. It is not unlikely that the method is referred to by Antyllus in the passage beginning—ποτὲ μὲν καταπείρον-τες ποτὲ δὲ ἀναπείροντες φλεβοτοῦμεν (Oribasius, *Collect.* VII. x).

This passage describing the technique of phlebotomy has given rise to great and voluminous discussion (see Daremberg's Oribas. vol. ii. p. 776) from the fact that Antyllus goes on to state that we operate καταπείροντες—cutting inwards—in cases where the vessels are deep, and ἀναπείροντες—cutting outwards—where the vessels are superficial, and the advice has seemed to most commentators to be the reverse of what one would expect. The explanation seems to me to be simple. Superficial vessels are those which could be seen standing out on applying the fillet, and were to be divided by the method in vogue at the present day by transfixing the vessel through its middle and bringing the lancet outwards. The reason of this is that the danger of injuring important structures lying deep to the vein was well understood by the ancients. Thus Galen warns against wounding the nerve in phlebotomy of the median, the tendon of the biceps in phlebotomy of the scapulo-cephalic, the artery in dividing the basilic, and so on. But in opening deep-lying veins the method of transfixing was inapplicable, and the bone was cut boldly down upon till the issue of blood showed that the vein was opened. The deep vessels which were divided were those about the scalp, and as they had no important relations they were divided by cutting through everything overlying the bone, often with razor-shaped knives. Thus Paulus Aegineta (VI. vii) says: 'When many deep vessels send a copious defluxion to the eyes we have recourse to the operation called Periscyphismus.' This consisted in making a transverse incision down to the bone over the vertex from one temple to the other.

The ' Katias.'

Κατιάς -ιάδος (ἡ) (Soranus, II. xviii) ; καθιάς (Paul, VI. lxxiv) ; κατιάδιον (τό) (Aetius, II. iii. 2) ; κατειάδιον (τό) (Aretaeus, *Cur. Morb. Diut.* i. 2).

In Soranus (Bib. II. xviii. par. 59, p. 359, ed. Rose) there occurs mention of an instrument for puncturing the membranes where they do not rupture spontaneously :

Χόριον δὲ μὴ ἀναστομούμενον κατιάδι προσεχόντως διαιρεῖν τῷ δακτύλῳ προκοιλάναντα τι μέρος.

The Latin version of Moschion has :

Folliculum verum non ruptum ante digito impresso formantes locum phlebotomo sollicite dividimus omnibus praedictis post encymatismis utimur (xviii. 10, p. 83, ed. Rose).

However, we cannot accept this as conclusive evidence that the katias was the same as the phlebotome, as I have already pointed out that this version of Moschion is a late retranslation into Latin of a Greek translation of the original Moschion. While the meagre references to the katias point to its having been a similar instrument to the phlebotome, it is by no means certain that the instruments were identical. The next writer who notices the instrument is Aretaeus, who mentions it in the cure of headaches (*Cur. Morb. Diut.* i. 2) :

' We abstract blood from the nostrils, and for this purpose push into them a long instrument named κατειάδιον, or the one called the scoop ' (τορύνη).

In a note to his edition of Celsus, Lee says Aretaeus ' invented an instrument having at the end a blade of grass, or made like a blade of grass, which was thrust into the nostrils to excite an haemorrhage in some affections of the head. This instrument is named κατειάδιον, from κατά and εἴα a blade of grass '.

I have shown, however, that Soranus, who wrote a century before Aretaeus, used the term, and a comparison of the various forms in which the word appears seems to me to point rather to a connexion with καθίημι, one meaning of which is ' to let blood '. The next writer who mentions it is Aetius (II. iii. 2, and again II. iv. 14), where he refers to its use in opening quinsy, in a chapter copied from Leonidas :

'If the patient be adult make him sit down, and, opening his mouth, depress the tongue with a spatula or a tongue depressor, and open the abscess with a scalpel or katias' (σμιλαρίῳ ἢ κατιάδι).

Paul says that abscess of the womb is to be exposed with a speculum and opened with a scalpel or katias (σπαθίῳ ἢ κατιάδι). Paul also refers to it in perforating the foetal cranium in delivery obstructed through hydrocephaly (πολυπικῷ σπαθίῳ ἢ καθιάδι ἢ σκολοπομαχαιρίῳ) (VI. lxxiv).

These somewhat scanty materials, summed up, give us the following results. We find the instrument used for opening the chorion, opening abscess of the womb, perforating the foetal cranium, drawing blood from the inside of the nose, and opening abscess of the tonsil. It cannot have been a needle, as Adams and Cornarius translate it, as some of these applications (e. g. perforating the foetal cranium) could not have been performed with a needle. The uses to which the instrument was put correspond very closely to the uses of the phlebotome, and from this and from the etymological significance of the word I am inclined to think that if it is not identical with the phlebotome it is at least only a variety of that instrument, with a handle longer than usual in order to adapt it for uterine and intranasal operations.

Spathion and Hemispathion.

Greek, σπαθίον (diminutive of σπάθη), ἡμισπάθιον ; Latin, spatha.

On several occasions a knife called σπαθίον is mentioned. Paul (VI. lxxiii) says of abscess of the womb :

'When the abscess is explored, if it is soft (and this may be ascertained by touching it with the finger) it is to be opened with a spathion or a needle knife' (σπαθίῳ ἢ κατιάδι).

Again, Paul (VI. lxxviii) says :

Find the orifice of the fistula, pass an ear probe through

it and cut down upon it. Divide the whole fistula with a hemispathion or a fistula-knife (ἡμισπαθίῳ ἢ σπαθίῳ συριγγοτόμῳ).

What the nature of the σπαθίον was, if indeed it was a distinct instrument and not a term for scalpels in general, we cannot definitely say. The etymology of the word would indicate a blade of the shape of a weaver's spattle, the two edges running into one at the point. Heister (i. 651) and Rhodius (Commentar. in *Scrib. Larg.* p. 46) agree in making the spathion a large two-edged scalpel, as also does Scultetus, who says of it :

Scalpellum ancipitem esse utrimque acutum et in superiore parte paulo latum, qui in extremitate sua in unam cuspidem coiret (*Arm. Chir.* Tab. II, fig. 1).

We shall see that one variety of spathion—that for detaching nasal polypus—was certainly of this shape.

Rhodius (loc. cit.) says the hemispathion is a small variety of the spathion.

An instrument in the Louvre has two blades of this shape at either end of a round handle ornamented with rolling grooves (Pl. VIII, fig. 8).

Polypus Knife.

Greek, πολυπικὸν σπαθίον, πολυποδικὸν σπαθίον ; Latin, *ferramentum acutum modo spathae factum.*

Paulus Aegineta (VI. xxv) thus describes the excision of nasal polypus :

'Holding in his right hand the polypus scalpel, which is shaped like a myrtle leaf and sharp pointed (πολυπικῷ σπαθίῳ τῷ μυρσινοειδεῖ ἀκμαίῳ), we cut round the polypus or fleshy tumour, applying the point of the steel blade (τὴν ἀκμὴν τοῦ σιδήρου) to the part where it adheres to the nose. Afterwards turning the instrument end for end (ἀντιστρέψαντες) we bring out the separated fleshy body with the scoop' (τῷ κυαθίσκῳ).

This description reminds us very forcibly of Celsus's account of the operation :

Ferramento acuto modo spathae facto, resolvere ab osse

oportet. Ubi abscissus est unco ferramento extrahendus est (VII. x).

These passages, especially that from Paul, show that like the majority of Roman instruments the polypus scalpel was a double instrument, with a sharp-pointed leaf-shaped blade at one end and a scoop at the other. The fact that it was able to work inside the nose shows that it could not have been of any great breadth. Paul says it was able to be used in the auditory canal.

'If there be a fleshy excrescence it may be excised with a pterygium knife or the polypus scalpel' (VI. xxiv).

This shows that it was less than a quarter of an inch broad at the most. It was used for several other purposes. Soranus refers to it for opening the foetal head in cranioclasis :—

Εἰ δὲ μείζονος τοῦ κεφαλίου ὑπάρχοντος ἡ σφήγωσις ἀποτελοῖτο, διὰ τοῦ ἐμβρυοτόμου ἢ τοῦ πολυπικοῦ σπαθίου κρυπτομένου μεταξὺ λιχανοῦ καὶ τοῦ μακροῦ δακτύλου κατὰ τὴν ἔνθεσιν (xviii. 63).

Paul copies this (VI. lxxiv). Soranus also says it may be used for dividing the membranes where they delay in rupturing.

There are two instruments of steel which are of the form indicated above. One is in the Museum of Montauban (Tarne - et - Garonne). The other was found at Vieille-Toulouse and is shown in Pl. VIII, fig. 1.

Lithotomy Knife.

Greek, λιθοτόμον (τό); Latin, scalpellus.

In describing lithotomy Paul says:

'We take the instrument called the lithotomy knife (τὸ καλούμενον λιθοτόμον), and between the anus and the testicles, not however in the middle of the perinaeum, but on one side, towards the left buttock, we make an oblique incision cutting down straight on the stone where it projects' (VI. lx).

Celsus, whose description of the operation is famous, gives us no more hint of the shape of the lithotomy knife than

Paul does. He only says 'multi hic scalpello usi sunt', and as he uses 'scalpellus' to denote all sorts of different knives, we can draw no information from that term. We may note, however, that both Celsus and Paul describe the operation as being performed by fixing the stone by means of the left index finger inserted in the anus, and cutting down directly upon it with one stroke as in opening an abscess. Now this sort of incision was always performed by early surgeons with a two-edged scalpel sharp at the point, and a knife of this sort was used for lithotomy by the Arabian surgeons, and after them by European surgeons down to comparatively recent times. Heister, for instance, shows as a lithotomy knife a large knife, like a phlebotome in shape. It is most likely, therefore, that the Greeks and Romans used a knife of this shape also.

A passage in Rufus of Ephesus shows that in his time the lithotomy knife had the handle shaped like a hook to extract the stone after the perineal incision was made :

Καὶ εἰ μὲν πρόχειρος εἴη, τῇ λαβῇ τοῦ μαχαιρίου ἐκβάλλειν, πεπιεσμένον δὲ τῇ λαβῇ τραχείᾳ τε καὶ καμπύλῃ ἐξ ἄκρου, ὡς ἂν μάλιστα συμφέροι τῷ ἔργῳ.

'And if it (the stone) be at hand we must eject it with the handle of the knife, made with the handle roughened and curved at the tip, as best suited for the operation' (ed. cit. p. 52).

One of the knives in the scalpel box shown in Pl. IV has the handle of this curved shape.

Although Celsus gives us no information about the shape of the ordinary lithotomy knife, he goes on to describe in detail a special variety of lithotomy knife invented by Meges, a surgeon of whom he had a very high opinion. As this passage has given rise to much discussion I shall quote Celsus's description in full :

Multi hic quoque scalpello usi sunt. Meges (quoniam is infirmior est potestque in aliquam prominentiam incidere, incisoque super illam corpore qua cavum subest, non secare sed relinquere quod iterum incidi necesse sit) ferramentum fecit rectum, in summa parte labrosum, in ima semicirculatum acutumque. Id receptum inter duos digitos, indicem ac medium, super pollice imposito, sic deprimebat ut simul cum carne si quid ex calculo prominebat incideret, quo consequabatur ut semel quantum satis esset aperiret (VII. xxvi).

'Here many have used the scalpel. Meges (since it is rather weak and may cut down upon some projecting part, and while the tissues overlying that are divided it may not divide those where there is a hollow underneath, but may leave a portion which requires to be divided afterwards) made an instrument straight, with a projecting lip at the heel and rounded and cutting at the tip. This, held between the two fingers, index and middle, the thumb being placed on the top, he pushed down so as to divide not only tissues but any projecting portion of the calculus, and as a consequence at one stroke he made a sufficient opening.'

Etangs in his edition of Celsus gives as his idea of the instrument described an instrument of the shape indicated in the accompanying diagram (Pl. VIII, fig. 6). Thus he makes the cutting edge a concave semicircle, and therefore we may dismiss his conjecture, for a cutting edge on this principle would never cut its way into the bladder in the manner described by Celsus.

Daremberg (*Gaz. Med. de Paris*, 1847, p. 163, &c.) conjectures an instrument which seems to me to be nearer the true interpretation (Pl. VIII, fig. 4). This instrument, with some modification, I would accept. The lunated handle figured by Daremberg is not strictly speaking what is meant by *labrosum*, and *summa parte* I take to refer to the back part of the blade, and not to the back part of the instrument as a whole. *Rectum* I take to indicate that the instrument was straight and not a curved bistoury. I conceive that the lithotomy knife of Meges was only a modification of the one in general use, and that in order to enable it to be held more firmly in the manner described by Celsus, Meges raised a lip on the handle at the heel of the blade, and in order to allow it to cut its way into the stone itself to some extent (which was his avowed object) he rounded the end of the blade, so that it might be rocked upon the stone without chipping as a pointed blade would do. I think the above explanation provides an instrument corresponding to a legitimate interpretation of the text and at the same time suited for the operation indicated (Pl. VIII, fig. 5).

Perforator for the foetal cranium.

Greek, ἐμβρυοτόμον.

A special instrument for perforating the foetal cranium is mentioned by Soranus (II. viii. p. 366):

Εἰ δὲ μείζονος τοῦ κεφαλίου ὑπάρχοντος ἡ σφήνωσις ἀποτελοῖτο, διὰ τοῦ ἐμβρυοτόμου ἢ τοῦ πολυπικοῦ σπαθίου κρυπτομένου μεταξὺ λιχανοῦ καὶ τοῦ μακροῦ δακτύλου κατὰ τὴν ἔνθεσιν.

'If the head be too big, the obstruction may be removed by the embryotome, or the polypus knife, concealed between the index finger and the thumb during its introduction.'

The other authors who recommend this unpleasant operation use mostly the polypus-scalpel or the phlebotome, and hence we may conjecture that a straight two-edged blade was considered the most suitable. The embryotome figured by Albucasis is of this shape (Pl. VIII, fig. 7), as is also the cutting part of the perforators of more modern times—fortunately now obsolete.

Probe pointed blade with two cutting edges.

There is in the Orfila Museum, Paris, a fine little two-edged bistoury of bronze with a probe point (Pl. VIII, fig. 2). It is a relic of the Roman occupation of Egypt. Its use must remain a matter of conjecture as we have no written description of such an instrument. It is perhaps a fistula knife.

II A. (a) Curved bistoury—'Crow Bill.'

Greek, ὀξυκόρακον σμίλιον.

In extirpating warts Paul (VI. lxxxvii) says we put them on the stretch with a vulsella and extirpate them radically with a scalpel shaped like a crow's beak or a phlebotome

(ὀξυκοράκῳ σμιλίῳ ἢ φλεβοτόμῳ ἐκ ῥιζῶν ἐξελεῖν). This un-
doubtedly refers to a curved scalpel, for the grappling
hook was called κόραξ.

In Celsus the instrument appears under the term *corvus*.
In describing the opening of the scrotal sac in the operation
for the radical cure of hernia he says :

Deinde eam ferramento, quod a similitudine corvum
vocant, incidere sic ut intrare duo digiti, index et medius,
possint (VII. xix).

Vulpes (Tav. VII, 3 and 4) figures two curved bistouries
from the Naples Museum. They have lost their tips. Both
are of the same shape, but one has the blade slightly larger
than the other. The handles are of bronze, the blades of
steel. A good example is seen in the Athens scalpel box
(Pl. IV).

A powerful variety so strongly curved as to resemble a
small billhook was found in the Roman hospital at Baden
(Pl. IX, fig. 5). The handle is of ivory, the blade is of steel,
and there is a mounting of bronze.

Pterygium Knife.

Greek, πτερυγοτόμος ὁ ; Latin, *scalpellus*.

Paul (VI. xviii), quoting Aetius, II. iii. 60, says that there
were two methods of curing pterygium. In the first the
pterygium was raised by a small sharp hook, and a needle
carrying a horsehair and a strong flaxen thread was passed
under it. Tension being made on the thread by an assistant,
the operator sawed off the pterygium towards the apex by
means of the horsehair. The base of the pterygium was then
severed with the scalpel for the plastic operation on entropion. The second method consisted in dissecting away the
pterygium (stretched as aforesaid with a thread) with the
instrument called the pterygotome (πτερυγοτόμῳ) care being
taken not to injure the lids.

Aetius (II. iii. 74) says that adhesion of the sclerotic to
the lid may be separated by means of the pterygotome.
Paul (VI. xxii) in empyema of the lachrymal sac dissects

out the part between the sac and the canthus with the pterygotome, and again in excision of polypus aurium he says it may be employed. These uses of the pterygotome point to its having been a sharp-pointed knife of a small size. Albucasis, who conveys entire the passage on pterygium from Paul, gives figures of both these instruments. The pterygotome which Albucasis depicts is a small, narrow, sharp-pointed scalpel (Pl. IX, fig. 2).

Knife for plastic operation on the eyelid.

Greek, ἀναρραφικὸν σμιλίον.

I have in describing the pterygotome given one instance of the use of the ' scalpel for the plastic operation ', viz. to dissect away the base of a pterygium the rest of which had been separated off by means of sawing with a horsehair. The plastic operation for entropion seems to have been one which was very frequently required. We know that granular ophthalmia with trichiasis as a sequela was very rife. Aetius (quoting from Leonidas) and Paul give very nearly the same account of the operation to remedy the trichiasis. Paul says :

' Having placed the patient on a seat either before us or on the left hand, we turn the upper eyelid outwards, and if it has long hairs we take hold of them between the index finger and thumb of the left hand ; but if they are very short we push a needle having a thread through the middle of the tarsus from within outwards. Then stretching the eyelid with the left hand by means of this thread, with the point of the scalpel held in the right hand, having everted the eyelid, behind the thread we make the inferior incision inside the hairs which irritate the eye, extending from the larger canthus to the smaller along the tarsus. After the inferior incision, having extracted the thread and having put a small compress under the thumb of the left hand, we stretch the eyelid upwards. Then arranging other small compresses on the canthi at their extremities we direct the assistant, who stands behind, to stretch the eyelid by means of them. Then by means of the ' scalpel for the plastic operation ' (ἀναρραφικοῦ σμιλίου) we make the first incision called the ' arrow-shaped ' a little above the hairs which are normal, extending from canthus to canthus and penetrating only the depth of the skin.   Afterwards we make the incision called the crescent-shaped, beginning at the same place as the former and carrying it upwards to such a height as to enclose the whole superabundant skin and ending in like manner as it did.   Thus the whole skin within the incision will have the shape of a myrtle leaf.   Having perforated the angle of this portion with a hook we dissect away the whole skin.   Then washing away the clots with a sponge we unite the lips of the incision with three or four sutures' (VII. viii).

The use of the scalpel for the plastic operation, therefore, was to make an incision in the eyelid in such a way as to enclose a leaf-shaped area and to dissect off the skin surrounded by the incision.   Albucasis figures it as a small but fairly broad blade with a rounded cutting tip (Pl. IX, fig. 3).

It must have been a small scalpel to suit the operation described, and to make the dissection indicated it must have been sharp-pointed.   It is contrasted to some extent with the pterygotome by Paul, and we saw that the pterygotome was narrow and sharp-pointed.   These various references to its use are in agreement with the supposition that it was of the shape figured by Albucasis.   I have considered it here because the question of its shape is rather hypothetical, and therefore it seemed best to consider it close by its confrere the pterygotome.   We may recall the fact that in the grave of the third-century oculist Severus several tiny scalpel handles were found.   These were probably handles for these two ophthalmic scalpels, but unfortunately only a trace of the steel remains.   Védrènes, in his edition of Celsus, figures an instrument from Pompeii of a shape which we are accustomed to associate with eye work (Pl. IX, fig. 6).

Uvula Knife.

Greek, σταφυλοτόμον.
This is a special scalpel for throat work, of whose shape

we know nothing. It is mentioned by Paul as a special scalpel for excision of the uvula :

'Wherefore, having seated the patient in the sunlight and directed him to gape wide, we seize with the uvula forceps or a common tenaculum upon the elongated part and drag it downwards and excise it with the instrument called the uvula knife (σταφυλοτόμῳ), or the scalpel used for the plastic operation on the eyelid ' (VI. xxxi).

The knife figured by Albucasis as used for the purpose is a small curved bistoury (Pl. IX, fig. 4). We have no other means of determining its shape. I have placed it here because it was mentioned along with the ' scalpel for the operation on the eyelid '.

Blade curved on the flat.—Tonsil Knife.

Greek, ἀγκυλοτόμον (ἀγκύλη, ' bend of elbow,' or ἀγκύλος, ' crooked ').

This instrument is described by Paul (VI. xxx) in the operation for removing the tonsils :

'Wherefore, having seated the patient in the sunlight, and directed him to open his mouth, one assistant holds his head and another presses down the tongue with a tongue depressor. We take a hook and perforate the tonsil with it and drag it outwards as much as we can without dragging the capsule out along with it, and then we cut it off by the root with the tonsillotome (ἀγκυλοτόμον) suited to that hand, for there are two such instruments having opposite curvatures. After the excision of one we may operate on the other in the same way.'

This passage clearly proves that there were two scalpels of a set, each having opposite curvatures after the manner of our right and left vesicovaginal fistula knives.

Curved blade cutting on one side, blunt-pointed.—Fistula Knife.

Greek, συριγγοτόμον, from σῦριγξ, ' a fistula.'

This was a falciform blade whose end was blunt, but the handle end was prolonged into a slender, rounded sound-like portion with a sharp point (Pl. IX, fig. 1). The narrow point was passed into a fistula, caught, and the whole instrument pulled outwards by means of it, thus dividing the overlying tissues with the falciform blade. This instrument remained in use till comparatively recent times. Heister figures a large number of varieties, and from him I have taken the figure shown, although it is also described and figured by Fabricius. The two following passages, taken in conjunction with each other, show that the classical instrument was of the form I have indicated. The first passage, from Galen, shows that the end of the blade was blunt, and that there was only one cutting side. The second, from Paul, shows that the blade was falciform and was operated in the manner I have stated. Galen (x. 415) says that in enlarging an abdominal wound we use a fistula knife (συριγγοτόμῳ). 'But the scalpels which are two-edged or have a point are distinctly to be avoided' (τὰ δ' ἀμφήκη τῶν μαχαιρίων ἢ κατὰ τὸ πέρας ὀξέα παντὶ τρόπῳ φευκτέα).

Secondly, Paul (VI. lxxviii) says:

'Having perforated the bottom of the fistula with the point of the falciform part of the syringotome (τοῦ δρεπάνου τοῦ συριγγοτόμου) bring the instrument out of the anus and so divide all the intervening space with the edge of the falciform part' (τῇ ἀκμῇ τοῦ δρεπάνου).

Another passage in the same chapter indicates that some of the syringotomes had an eye in the instrument:

Τινὲς δὲ ἐν τῷ τρήματι τοῦ συριγγιακοῦ δρεπάνου τὸ λίνον ἐνείραντες.

There was also a straight variety of the instrument (τὰ καλούμενα ὀρθὰ συριγγοτόμα, Paul, VI. lii).

Curved blade cutting on two edges.

A curved blade of a somewhat unusual type is described by Galen in discussing the dissection of the thorax (ii. 673). However, the description is unmistakably clear. He says:

Χρῆσθαι δ' αὐτῆς μάλιστα τῷ κυρτῷ μέρει κεχαλκευμένης ὁμοίως ἑκατέρωθεν, ὥστε ἀμφικύρτους ἔχειν ἀμφοτέρας τὰς τεμνούσας γραμμὰς ἀλλὰ κατὰ μὲν τὴν ἑτέραν σιμῆς, κατὰ δὲ τὴν ἀντικειμένην ταύτῃ κυρτῆς.

' It is best to have the curved part forged alike on both sides so that the cutting edges are curved in two ways, viz. one concave and the other convex.'

A smaller variety for fine dissection is referred to in the same book (εἰς ὅπερ ἐστὶν ἐπιτηδειοτάτη μυρσίνη κυρτή, ii. 674).

Shears.

Greek, ψαλίς ; Latin, forfex.

Oribasius treats of cutting the hair as a regular medical procedure, in a special chapter, περὶ κουρᾶς καὶ ξυρήσεως. Celsus also frequently refers to cutting the hair as a therapeutic measure. Possibly the ancients found difficulty in putting an edge sufficiently smooth for surgical purposes on their shears. We have a few references to the use of the shears for cutting tissues. Celsus, in the treatment of abdominal injury with protusion of omentum, says :

Omentum quoque considerandum est: ex quo, si quid iam nigri et emortui est, forfice excidi debet: si integrum est, leniter super intestina deduci (VII. xvi).

Again in the operation for the radical cure of hernia he says :

Fuerunt etiam qui omentum forfice praeciderent: quod in parvulo non est necessarium ; si maius est, potest profusionem sanguinis facere, siquidem omentum quoque venis quibusdam etiam maioribus illigatum est. Neque vero, si discisso ventre id prolapsum forfice praeciditur, quum et emortuum sit et aliter tutius avelli non possit, inde huc exemplum transferendum est (VII. xxi) :

' There have been others who cut away the omentum with scissors, which is unnecessary if the portion is small ; and if very great it may occasion a profuse haemorrhage, since the omentum is connected with some of even the largest veins. But this objection cannot be applied in cases where, the belly being cut open, the prolapsed omentum is removed with shears, since it may be both gangrenous and unable to be removed in any other way with safety.'

We have also two references in Paulus Aegineta. He says some of the moderns effect a cure of warty excrescences on the penis by a pair of shears (ψαλίδι, VI. lviii), and dealing with relaxation of the scrotum he says that Antyllus, having first transfixed the superfluous skin with three or four ligatures, cut off what was external to them with a pair of sharp-pointed shears or a scalpel (ψαλίδι ἐπάκμῳ ἢ σμίλῃ), and having secured the parts with sutures he effected healing with the treatment for recent wounds.

Shears are very common objects in museums. Some are of bronze and some are of steel. Judging from the relative numbers in which they have been preserved it would seem that the steel shears far outnumbered the bronze. In Pl. X, fig. 5 is shown a bronze pair from the Naples Museum, found in Pompeii.

CHAPTER IV

PROBES

GREEK, μήλη, κοπάριον, ὑπάλειπτρον, ὑπαλειπτρίς; Latin, *specillum*.

This is a very comprehensive class. The original specillum was no doubt a simple sound. Varro thus defines the specillum : ' Quo oculos inunguimus quibus specimus specillum est. Graecis μήλη dicitur.' Thus it meant a probe or sound.

μήλη is probably derived from μῆλον, an apple or fruit, from the olivary enlargement at the end of a sound.

The term ὑπάλειπτρον, which is frequently used by Hippocrates, originally meant an ointment spatula, being derived from ὑπαλείφω, to spread ointment. But the custom of combining two instruments on one shaft gradually led to the application of these terms, especially the term specillum, to denote a large variety of instruments.

The name κοπάριον is evidently derived from the resemblance of the probe to the pestle, which was such a frequent utensil in Greek homes. It is connected with κόπανον, 'pestle,' κοπανιστήριον, ' mortar,' and κοπανίζω, ' bray,' and κοπτάριον, a medicament pounded in a mortar (Dioscorides, iv. 190). The exact significance of the term κοπάριον is sometimes difficult to determine. It is easy to prove that in general it is merely a sound. Thus Paul (VI. lxxviii), in quoting a passage from Hippocrates, substitutes κοπάριον for the word μήλη, which Hippocrates uses to denote the sound used for exploring a fistula. Throughout this chapter, in which the word occurs ten times in all, Briau translates it by ' manche du scalpel ', although the whole context shows that a probe is meant. Even where it is spoken of as an eyed

probe (διὰ τετρημένου κοπαρίου) Briau translates it by 'au
moyen du manche percé d'un scalpel', an expression which
is meaningless to a surgeon. Briau evidently thinks it is
derived from κόπτω, and at times it seems as if it might denote a cutting instrument. Thus Adams, in a note to Paul,
VI. lxxvii, says, ' if the κοπάριον, however, was the same as the
μήλη or specillum it was evidently used for cutting with, as
well as for cutting upon ', and on one occasion (Paul, VI. lxxx)
he translates κοπάριον by ' knife '. Liddell and Scott translate
it as 'a small knife'. A careful examination of those
passages where it seems to indicate a cutting instrument
will show, however, that only blunt dissection, which was
frequently performed with the spatula end of a probe, is
meant. I am quite convinced that the word κοπάριον is only
a late Greek term for the earlier μήλη, and means essentially
a sound, and not a knife. While on this subject we may
note that throughout the codices and texts there is great
confusion between words meaning probe and words meaning
scalpel. The proper forms σμίλη, ' scalpel,' and μήλη, ' probe,'
are distinct, but the inferior reading σμήλη is frequent in
both codices and texts as a bastard, for σμίλη is often written
σμήλη incorrectly, and μήλη often becomes σμήλη, just as
μικρός is written σμικρός. Thus in Paul (VI. viii), where the
author is describing the eversion of the eyelid by means of
the olivary point of a probe (τῷ πυρῆνι τῆς μήλης), four codices
and the Aldine and Basle texts read σμήλης, two codices read
σμύλης, one reads μήλης, four μίλης, and Briau reads σμίλης.
In a case like this only a knowledge of surgery can tell us
whether a probe or scalpel is meant.

The Specillum as a Sound.

The ancients were fully aware of the value of the information to be gained by searching the recesses of a lesion with
a rod of metal. Celsus (v. 28) says regarding fistulae:

Ante omnia autem demitti specillum in fistulam convenit,
ut quo tendat et quam alte perveniat scire possimus; simul
etiam protinus humida an siccior sit: quod extracto specillo

patet. Si vero os in vicino est id quoque disci potest si iam
necne eo fistula penetraverit et quatenus nocuerit; nam si
molle est quod ultimo specillo contingitur, intra carnem
adhuc vitium est, si magis id renititur, ad os ventum est.
Ibi deinde si labitur specillum, nondum caries est: si non
labitur sed aequali innititur, caries quidem, verum adhuc
levis est: si inaequale quoque et asperum subest, vehementius
os exesum est. At cartilago ubi subsit, ipsa sedes docet;
perventumque esse ad eam ex renisu patet.

'But first it is well to put a probe into the fistula to learn
where it goes and how deeply it reaches, also whether it
is moist or rather dry as is evident when the probe is withdrawn. Further, if there be bone adjacent, it is possible to
learn whether the fistula has entered it or not and how
deeply it has caused disease. For if the part is soft which
is reached by the end of the probe the disease is still inter-
muscular; if the resistance be greater it has reached the
bone: if there the probe slip there is as yet no caries. If it
does not slip but meets with a uniform resistance there is
indeed caries, but it is as yet slight. If what is below is
uneven and rough the bone is seriously eroded, and whether
there is cartilage below will be known by the situation, and
if the disease has reached it will be evident from the
resistance.'

These remarks show that with the probe the ancients had
cultivated the tactus eruditus to a high degree, and the
remarks of Aetius and Paul are equally to the point.

The tips of the probes which have survived vary considerably in size and shape. Some have a point which is almost
sharp like a stylet; in others the natural thickness of the
shaft is kept right to the tip, which is simply rounded
off or there is an oval enlargement like that on our
olivary probes and sounds. In rare cases the enlargement
is globular. The oval enlargement was named by the
Greeks πυρήν, which means 'olive-kernel'. The sixteenth-
century translators uniformly render this by 'nucleus', which
is a convenient term to use, but it has no classical Latin
authority. Indeed, there is no classical Latin equivalent
used by medical authors. Theodorus Priscianus uses *baca*
(*sic*), a berry, and *bacula*, little berry, and in the *Additamenta*

(I. viii. 21, ed. Rose) he uses the transliteration *pyrena meles*. But this is African Latin.

A probe without enlargement at the tip was called ἀπυρηνομήλη or ἀπυρομήλη. The ear probe is frequently referred to as belonging to this class. These probes without nuclei were specially adapted for wrapping round with wool to apply medicaments, or wipe away discharge.

The size of the nucleus varied in different varieties of probe, but was pretty constant in each particular. It was largest in the probe known as the spathomele—a combination of spatula and probe which was in extremely common use for pharmaceutical purposes. The nucleus of this probe was such a well-known object that it is frequently referred to as a standard of size and shape. Galen (ii. 898) says:

' In the cervix uteri is the foramen by which the woman both passes the monthly flux and receives the semen of the husband. By it also the foetus leaves the womb. It is marvellous how it varies in size according to circumstances. When the woman is not pregnant it admits the nucleus of a probe or something slightly larger' (πυρῆνα μὲν μήλης ἐπιδέχεται ἢ βραχύ τι τούτου παχύτερον).

Here Kühn translates πυρῆνα by ' acuminatum capitulum specilli', which is incorrect. It is an olivary enlargement, not sharp point. In Paul (VI. xc), we have the nucleus given at the measure of distance between the perforations by which a bone was surrounded preparatory to its excision by means of chisels: ' the space between the perforations made by the drills should be the breadth of the nucleus of a probe' (τὸ μῆκος πυρῆνος).

Aetius (III. i. 16) says in volvulus the sphincter ani is so contracted that the nucleus of a probe cannot be got in.

Paul (VI. xxi) says that in couching a cataract we must enter the couching needle a nucleus breadth from the iris.

Besides its use as a sound the nucleus was frequently used as a means of applying medicaments, either in the form of ointments or dry powder, to affected parts.

Paul (VI. ix) says that in the cases of entropion, where the ordinary plastic operation is objected to, an elliptical piece may be burnt out of the eyelid with caustic applied on the nucleus of a probe (πυρηνοσμήλης), and similarly after removal of sebaceous cysts from the lid, levigated salts may be applied on the nucleus (τὸν πυρῆνα τῆς μήλης).

Aetius (II. iv. 23), quoting from Galen, says that in caries of the teeth some wax may be warmed on the nucleus of a probe (πυρῆνος μήλης), and again (II. iv. 14) he directs us to use it for application of pomade to the face (πυρῆνι μήλης). It would seem that this, and not the exploration of wounds, was the original use to which the olivary-pointed probe was put, for in early Egyptian tombs small pestle-like probes are, as a rule, found accompanying the toilet pigment boxes which are so common. They are mostly made of wood (Pl. X, fig. 2). The kohl-stick was not unknown to Greek ladies. (See Eustathius, *Comment. in Iliad.*)

Hitherto I have spoken of the probe as if it were a single instrument; but, as a matter of fact, the ends of the shaft are usually fashioned to serve different purposes. Thus at one end there will be a probe, at the other a spatula, a spoon, or a hook. Some of these combinations have names of their own, and others are so frequently met with that they too seem to have been constant types.

It may simplify matters if we anticipate a little and remark that while the uses of the probes in actual surgery were the same as at the present day, in the minor surgery, consisting of the application of medicaments and toilet preparations, they were used in a slightly different manner. Semi-solids, like eyebrow pigment and eye ointments, were applied on olivary-pointed probes. Liquids, like ear and eye drops, were usually instilled by squeezing a ball of wool dipped in the liquid and placed round the middle of a probe, and letting it run off the point. Thus a common form of toilet instruments consists of a probe-like instrument with an olive at one end and a sharp stylet at the other. Ligulae with scoops were used to withdraw drops of fluid essences,

&c. from unguentaria. Some of these ligulae run up to a foot and a half in length.

The specilla which remain to us are mostly made of bronze. A few are overlaid with gold and silver, and a few are solid gold or solid silver. We read, however, of specilla of lead, tin, copper, and wood, and of the use of a boar's bristle or a stalk of garlic for searching fistulae.

I shall now proceed to classify and discuss these different varieties, premising, however, that no hard and fast line can be drawn between different types. They shade off into each other by imperceptible gradations, so that whatever system of classification we adopt bastard forms are sure to occur.

Double Simple Probe.

Greek, ἀπυρηνομήλη, ἀπυρομήλη ; Latin, *specillum.*

The simplest form of specillum is a plain rod of metal rounded off at either end. These are not infrequently met with. I figure one from my collection. Its length is 14·5 cm., its diameter 2 mm. At either end it tapers rapidly off to a blunt point. At a distance of 3 cm. from one end is a raised ring (Pl. X, fig. 4). A similar probe in silver may be seen in the Musée de Cinquantenaire, Brussels. It was found with other probes in an étui. Pl. X, Fig. 3 shows a rather longer specimen from the Naples Museum. A variety with non-tapered ends is seen in Pl. X, fig. 1. It is also from the Naples Museum. Pl. XI, fig. 4 shows a probe, from my own collection, which carries the snake of Aesculapius at one end. One with a double snake (caduceus form) was found in the Roman Hospital at Baden (Pl. XI, fig. 2).

Specilla with two olivary ends.

Greek, διπύρηνος μήλη, ἀμφίσμιλος.

A slender sound with slight olivary enlargement at either end is very frequently mentioned under the name διπύρηνος μήλη by Galen. He also calls it ἀμφίσμιλος. Thus he says :

Καί σοι διχόθεν ἔστι διεμβάλλειν αὐτοῦ τι τῶν παρασκευασμένων
λεπτὸν εἴτε ἀμφίσμιλον, εἴτε διπύρηνον ὀνομάζειν ἐθέλεις, εἰ δέ τι
λεπτότερον δέῃ καὶ μηλωτίδα (ii. 581).

'And in the double passage you must insert some one of
the slender instruments you have at hand, either a double-
ended probe (a ' double olive ' if you prefer to call it so),
or if something finer be necessary, even an ear probe.'

In dealing with fistulae Paul (VI. lxxvii) says :

'We must first examine them with a sound if they be
straight, or with a very flexible 'double olive' (διπυρήνῳ
εὐκαμπεῖ), such as those made of tin or the smallest of those
made of bronze, if they be crooked.'

Paul refers to its use as a cautery to destroy the roots
of hairs after epilation (VI. xiv) :

'Some, preferring cauterizing to the operation of trans-
plantation, evert the eyelid, and with a cilia forceps dragging out the offending hair, or two or even three hairs,
apply a heated double-olive probe or an ear probe, or some
such slender instrument, to the place from which the hair
or hairs were removed' (Διαπυρίνον ἢ μηλωτίδα ἤ τι τοιοῦτον
λεπτὸν ὄργανον πεπυρωμένον εἴρουσι τῷ τόπῳ ὅθεν ἡ θρὶξ ἢ αἱ τρίχες
ἐκομίσθησαν).

Here Briau reads πυρῆνα (an olivary point), but the
balance of the evidence of the codices is in favour of
διαπυρίνον, and the parallel to the passage quoted from Galen
is so complete that I have no hesitation in adopting the
reading given above.

I give an example of the dipyrene from my own collection.
It is 11·2 cm. long. The shaft is unequally divided by
a ringed fluting into two portions ; 4·5 cm. and 6·7 cm. long
respectively. The shorter portion of the shaft is plain, the
longer is grooved longitudinally by eight grooves (Pl. XI,
fig. 1). In many instances the dipyrene carried an eye in
one of its olives. This variety is frequently mentioned.
Thus Paul (VI. xxv) says, under treatment of nasal polypus :

'Taking then a thread moderately thick like a cord, and
having tied knots on it at the distance of two or three
finger-breadths, we introduce it into the eye of a dipyrene

(διπυρήνου τρήματι), and we push the other end of the probe (τὸ ἕτερον πέρας τοῦ διπυρήνου) upwards to the ethmoid openings, withdrawing it by the palate and the mouth, and then pulling with both hands we, as it were, saw the fleshy bodies away by means of the knots.'

Pl. XI, figs. 5 and 3 show single olive probes for the application of semi-solid medicaments. The former is from the outfit of the oculist of Rheims, in the Museum at St-Germain-en-Laye ; the latter, more highly ornamented by spirally twisting the stem, is from my own collection.

Spathomele or Spatula probe.

Greek, ὑπάλειπτρον, σπαθομήλη ; Latin, spathomele (Theodorus Priscianus), spathomela (Marcellus) ; German, Spatelsonde.

Almost every medical writer mentions the spathomele. It consists of a long shaft with an olivary point at one end and a spatula at the other. Galen (*Lex.*) calls the one στρόγγυλον μήλην, the other μήλη πλατεῖα. It was a pharmaceutical rather than a strictly surgical instrument. The olive end was used for stirring medicaments, the spatula for spreading them on the affected part or on lint. Galen (xiii. 466) says that certain applications are to be softened in the hand with rosaceum by means of the spathomele (μαλάξας ἐπὶ τῆς χειρὸς διὰ σπαθομήλης).

Marcellus frequently refers to it as used for stirring liquids in a vessel :

Immo manu vel digitis moderantibus paulatim insperges et adsidue spathomela commovebis et permiscebis, post haec omnia mittes oleum chamaemelinum, et iterum igni non nimio adposita olla lente et paulatim decoques medicamen, ita ut illud manu non contingas, sed spathomela agites (vii. 19).

In xiv. 44 he mentions a spathomele of copper :

Oportet autem moveri aquam ipsam rudicula vel spathomela aeris rubri.

The following passage from Theodorus Priscianus refers to its use for applying ointment to an affected part :

Si veluti carbunculus innatus fuerit, lycium cum melle contritum suppono frequenter per diem et spathomela temptante (*Euporiston*, xxvii).

Aetius (II. iv. 16) directs a particular medicament to be rubbed in and to be scraped off after a moderate space of time with a spathomele (τῇ σπαθομήλῃ).

The spathomele was used by painters for preparing and mixing their colours. The very large numbers in which they are found would indicate that their use was not confined to medical men.

Although the nucleus of the spathomele was too large to admit of its use as a probe for small lesions, it is evident that in exploring large cavities it must have been a valuable instrument. Galen (ii. 712) says:

' In small bodies the opening into the torcular Herophili may not be large enough to admit a spathomele nucleus, and therefore we must try some of the other olivary probes or even an ear probe, and cut alongside it.'

Priscianus alludes to plugging the nares with it :

Prius spathomeles extremo in baca molli lana obvoluto glebas sanguinis e naribus frequentius purgare nos convenit, post lana identidem obturando perclaudere (xiv).

' First of all we must frequently wipe away the clots of blood from the nose with the end of a spathomele wrapped on the ' berry' with soft wool, and then occlude it by plugging with wool in the same way.'

From Leonidas (Aetius, VI) we learn that it was used as a tongue depressor. He says :

' In inflammation of the throat in adults seat the patient, open his mouth and depress the tongue with a tongue depressor or a spathomele, and open the abscess with a scalpel or a needle-knife.'

The following passage from Galen shows that it was used as a substitute for the meningophylax (*q. v.*) :

' Having separated the pleura from the rib and placed a thin meningophylax or a flat spathomele (σπαθομήλην πλατεῖαν) between the ribs, and taking care that you neither tear nor perforate the membrane, which being properly accomplished, cut the bone of the rib with two chisels placed opposed to each other' (ii. 686).

Soranus (xxvii) refers to its use as a cautery:

'After cutting off the umbilical cord, cauterize the umbilicus with a heated reed, or the flat of a probe' (τοῦ πλάτεος τῆς μήλης).

An interesting passage in Aetius shows that it was used as a dissector in opening up an occluded vagina:

'Pass a sound into the cervix, and dissect with the spathomele below the spot marked out by the sound' (Aet. IV. iv. 96).

This probably means blunt dissection only, as none of the spathomeles found have edges sharp enough to be actually cutting. Large numbers of this instrument have been found. It is the commonest surgical instrument in museums. It must be remembered, however, that not every spathomele is a surgical instrument strictly speaking, as pharmacopolists and even artists used exactly similar instruments.

The average length of twenty specimens measured by me was 16 cm. Of this the nucleus occupies 1·5 cm., the spatula 6 cm. The average diameter of the nucleus is 7·5 mm. The width of the spatula averages 15 mm., but the size and shape of the spatula both vary considerably.

The different varieties of shape will be better understood by a reference to the accompanying figures of actual specimens than from a written description. Pl. XII, shows neatly formed specimens from various sources; the specimen shown in fig. 3 having ornamental grooves along the length of the shaft. Figs. 3 and 4, Pl. XIII show coarse, thick specimens, which are most likely to have been used for non-medical purposes. All have the characteristic oar-blade shape, though the outline varies greatly. In some the blade widens out at the end, so that the tip is broad and rounded. In others the blade slopes to a rounded point, or the point is quite acute. The edges of the blade are usually thick and blunt. In some specimens, however, the edges are thin, sharp, and almost suitable for use for cutting with. These are well adapted for use as blunt dissectors.

The shaft, as a rule, is plain, occasionally it is ornamented with longitudinal or spiral fluting. More rare is a silver band, inlaid in a spiral round the shaft. I have seen a few specimens which have been entirely plated with gold.

Hitherto I have taken no notice of spathomeles in which the spatulae are not flat. In many specimens, however, the blades are hollowed. For these it seems advisable to constitute a special class, which may be called the cyathiscomele class.

Cyathiscomele.

German, *Löffelsonde.*

Although this variety of the spathomele is not one which is specially mentioned by any classical writer, it is convenient to have a name by which we can denote that variety of the spathomele in which the blade is not flat.

It has the same large oval nucleus as the flat spathomele, and the same shaft, plain, or fluted, or overlaid with silver, but the spatula is replaced by a spoon, the outline of which shows the same variety of form as we met with in the spatula. The depth of the spoon varies greatly. Pl. XIV, fig. 3 shows an instrument in which the two lateral halves of the blade, instead of lying exactly in the same plane, meet in the midline at a slight angle so as to form a cavity obtusely angular on cross section, and gently rounded on longitudinal section :

Cross sec. . . .

Long. sec. . . .

Pl. XV, fig. 1 shows a similar arrangement, except that the cavity is more marked, and the tip instead of being sharp is rounded. In Pl. XIV, fig. 1 the cavity is so marked that a typical spoon is formed. This specimen is interesting as showing the ornamentation of the shaft by overlaying a spiral silver wire. It is from the Naples Museum, and it is figured by Vulpes. Other varieties are seen in Plates XIV,

XV. Pl. XV, fig. 4 shows a very coarse, thick specimen.
The scope of the cyathiscomele in medical art is evidently
like the flat spathomele to act occasionally as a sound, but
mainly to mix, measure, and apply medicaments.   Some
are adapted for use as curettes.   But the large number in
which this instrument occurs would of itself indicate that
it was used for lay as well as medical purposes.   Many are
toilet articles.   An interesting discovery of two typical
specimens in the grave of a lady artist was made in Vendée
in 1847.   Among a number of colour pots and alabaster
mortars for rubbing down and mixing colours was an étui
similar to the typical cylindrical instrument case of the
ancient surgeon, and in this were two spoon probes like
the one shown in Pl. XIV, fig. 1.   Evidently they were
favourite instruments of the painter, and had been used
by her for mixing and preparing her colours.[1]

The form of cyathiscomele, in which the two lateral halves
of the scoop meet at an angle (Pl. XIV, fig. 1), has a tendency
to split along the ridge in the middle of the scoop if
roughly handled.   One of these, to which this accident has
happened, is in the Naples Museum (Pl. XV, fig. 3) and has an
interesting history.   In 1847 Vulpes described it as a guard
for dividing the fraenum linguae, and successive writers
have copied this ever since, and it is so described in the
catalogue.   As the photograph shows, it is only a spoon
probe which had been trod on or otherwise damaged, and
which had split down the centre, or rather near the centre, for
the crack has deviated at its termination from the midline.
The termination of the notch thus formed has quite a different appearance from the figure by Vulpes.   The accident is
not an uncommon one.   There is in the Capitoline Museum
an instrument to which precisely the same has happened,
and I have a probe in my own possession which has split,
and which with a little manipulation would make a beautiful duplicate of the one in the Naples Museum (Pl. XV, fig.

---

[1] Blümner, *Technologie und Terminologie der Gewerbe und Künste bei
Griechen und Römern*, vol. iii. p. 458.

1). It is almost certain that the guard is quite a modern invention.

Many ancient writers point out the danger of wounding the vein, but none mention the guard. Thus Celsus says:

Horum extrema lingua vulsella prehendenda est, sub eaque membrana incidenda: magna cura habita ne venae quae iuxta sunt violentur et profusione sanguinis noceant (VII. xii).

Paul says:

' The patient is to be placed in a proper seat, the tongue is to be raised to the roof of the mouth and the membranous fraenum cut transversely. But if the curvature is occasioned by a cicatrix we transfix the callus by a hook and draw it upwards, and making a cross incision free the bent parts, taking care not to make deep incisions of the parts, for haemorrhages, which have been found difficult to stop, have thereby been occasioned' (VI. xxix).

Aetius gives a similar account.

These writers, then, all take note of the possibility of wounding the vein, but give no clue that they knew of the utility of a cloven plate in preventing the accident. Further, the Arabs, timid operators all and fond of describing safeguards such as this, give no mention of it, although Albucasis, Rhases, Avicenna, and Haly Abbas all describe the operation. I can find no reference to the use of a guard for this purpose until quite recent times.

Ear specillum.

Greek, μηλωτίς, -ίδος, μηλωτρίς, ἀπυρομήλη, τῇ πυρῆνα μὴ ἐχούσῃ τούτεστι τῇ μηλωτρίδι (Galen, Lexicon); ὠτογλυφίς, μήλην ἐξωτίδα (Galen, Lexicon); Latin, *oricularium specillum* (Celsus); *auriscalpium* (Scrib. Largus); German, *Ohrlöffel.*

Of all the specilla this is one of the most frequently mentioned by name. It consists of a small narrow scoop at one end and a simple probe without olivary enlargement at

the other. We shall discuss the scoop first. The following
passage from Archigenes describes it (Galen, xii. 652):

'If a bean, stone, &c., fall into the ear remove it with the
small narrow scoop of the ear specillum' (κναθίσκῳ στενῷ
μικρῷ μηλωτρίδος).

Again Galen (loc. cit.) and Paul (VI. xxiv) say that in
cases where foreign bodies cannot be got out of the
ear by more simple methods, we must incise behind the
ear and remove them by means of the ear scoop. The
removal of foreign bodies from the ear by means of this
instrument is very frequently referred to, and shows that
the scoop was small. Celsus says (VI. vii):

'When a person begins to experience a dullness of hearing,
which very often happens after long continued headaches,
first of all we must examine the ear itself, for there will
appear either a scab such as occurs upon ulcers, or a collection of sordes. If there is a scab it ought to be fomented
with warm oil or with verdigris in honey, or leek juice or
a little nitre in hydromel, and when the scabs have been
detached from the part, the ear is to be washed out with
tepid water, in order that being spontaneously separated it
may be the more easily extracted with the ear specillum
(oriculario specillo). If there is cerumen and it is soft, it
is to be extracted with the same specillum, or if it is hard
vinegar with a little water is to be put in, and when it is
softened the ear is to be washed out and evacuated in the
same way.'

In VI. vii he says:

Ubi vero vermes orti sunt, protrahendi oriculario specillo
sunt.

'Where worms have arisen they are to be extracted with
an ear specillum.'

Celsus also recommends it for extracting a calculus from
the meatus urinarius (VII. xxvi):

Eum, si fieri potest, oportet evellere vel oriculario specillo,
vel eo ferramento quo in sectione calculus protrahitur.

'It, if possible, is to be extracted with the specillum or
the instrument for extracting the calculus in lithotomy.'

Aetius (III. v) also describes removal of urethral calculus in this way.

The following passage from Paul (VI. xl) on venesection shows that in cases where the band of Antyllus could not be applied, the back of the ear scoop was pressed on the proximal end of the vein, in order to obstruct the flow of blood and cause it to discharge by the opening made with the phlebotome:

'Tie a ligature round the neck, and when the frontal vein is properly filled divide it with the point of a phlebotome or a scalpel. In the same way we open the external jugulars for chronic ophthalmia, producing a discharge of blood with the scoop of a probe' (κυαθίσκου μήλης).

Adams evidently misunderstood this passage. He translates it 'with the concave part of a scalpel', which is meaningless. This use of the scoop will also explain an otherwise obscure passage in Hippocrates (iii. 678). He says:

'In letting blood avoid pressing hard with the specillum (καὶ ὅταν ἀφαιρῇς τὸ αἷμα τῇ μήλῃ μὴ κάρτα πιέζειν ὡς μὴ φλάσις προσγίνηται) lest injury be caused.'

Of the use of the ear scoop as a curette we have several instances. Thus Aetius (II. iii. 81) recommends it for curetting the interior of a chalazion, and again (II. iii. 84), cf. Galen, *Comp. Med.* vii. 2. The scoop was also used for applying medicaments, especially to the eye. Liquid applications were poured from it, semi-solid were applied with the back of it (*averso specillo*). This use of the back of the scoop has often been misunderstood. The natural translation of the phrase *averso specillo* is 'with the probe turned away', i. e. the back of the probe. Scultetus, however (*Tab.* VIII. vii), considers that it refers to a spatula probe, and says it means the probe turned end for end. Other translators adopt this meaning. Deneffe (*Les Oculistes Gallo Romains*, p. 108), e. g., says:

Il faut entendre par *averso specillo* la partie de la spatule

opposée à celle qui sert comme sonde, c'est-à-dire son ex-
trémité large, l'autre bout étant le plus souvent olivaire.

Scribonius Largus puts the true meaning of the phrase
beyond doubt. He directs us, after the application of
caustic to haemorrhoids, to endeavour to get them to fall
off by the back of an ear scoop, which part the Greeks
called the spoon ('auriscalpio averso quam partem κυαθίσκον
Graeci vocant').

Marcellus copies this passage from Scribonius, but alters
it. He says: 'de specilli latitudine illinendae sunt' (xxxi.
6, p. 329).

I shall now proceed to give a few instances of this use of
the back of the scoop in minor surgical manipulations.

In ancyloblepharon Celsus says the eyelids are to be
separated with the back of the scoop.

Igitur aversum specillum inserendum, diducendaeque eo
palpebrae sunt (VII. vii. 6).

The back of the scoop was used as a retractor for delicate
structures. In radical cure of hernia Celsus directs us to
keep the bowel from prolapsing by means of it:

'For if the piece be small it is to be pushed back over the
groin into the abdomen, either with the finger or the back
of the specillum.'

Nam quod parvulum est super inguen in uterum vel
digito vel averso specillo repellendum est (VII. xxi).

In the cure of varicocele it is used to replace the veins in
position:

Tum venae, quaecunque protractae sunt, in ipsum inguen
averso specillo compelli debent (VII. xxii).

'Then the veins which have been drawn upon ought to
be replaced with the back of a specillum.'

In sloughing ulcer of the bladder it is used to separate
the lips of the perineal wound:

Quod si antequam vesica purgata est orae se glutina-
runt, dolorque et inflammatio redierunt, vulnus digitis vel
averso specillo diducendum est (VII. xxvii).

'But, if before the bladder has become cleansed the lips unite and pain and inflammation have returned, the wound is to be separated with the fingers or the back of a specillum.'

We shall next proceed to discuss the other end of the ear specillum. This was a simple probe. It had no nucleus. In his Lexicon Galen defines it thus:

'Απυρομήλη· τῇ πυρῆνα μὴ ἐχούσῃ τούτεστι τῇ μηλωτρίδι.

'Probe without olivary enlargement—that is to say " the ear specillum ".'

Not only was its tip not expanded into a nucleus, it was actually sharp. Galen (xiv. 787) treating of fistula in ano, says in non-perforating fistulae we perforate all the sound flesh with the sharp end of an ear probe (τῷ ὀξεῖ τῆς μηλωτίδος). The chief use of an ear probe in aural work was to instil liquids into the ear. A large ball of wool saturated with the liquid was wrapped round the middle of the probe, and on squeezing this the liquid ran down and dropped into the meatus. There are many mediaeval illustrations showing the ear probe used in this fashion. Sometimes, however, we read of the tip of the probe being wrapped in a small ball of wool, which was dipped in some sticky substance to extract foreign bodies from the ear. Galen (xii. 689) says foreign bodies may be removed thus by a probe dipped in resin.

The ear probe seems to have been much used for probing wounds and fistulae when a very slender instrument was required. Galen (ii. 581), in describing the torcular Herophili, says:

'And in the double passage you may be able to insert some of the slender instruments you have at hand, a double ended probe—a ' double-olivary ' if you prefer to call it so— or if something smaller be necessary even an ear specillum' (καὶ μηλωτρίδα).

In his chapter on the extraction of weapons (VI. lxxxviii) Paul says:

'If the weapon has a tang, which is ascertained by examination with an ear probe' (ἐκ τῆς μηλωτῆς).

As a cautery it was used to destroy the roots of hairs, which had been removed for trichiasis. Paul says:

' We may apply a double olive or an ear probe (μηλωτίδα) or some such fine instrument heated ' (VI. xiii).

In fistula in ano Paul says it may be used as a director to cut upon.

' Having introduced a sound or an ear probe (ὑποβάλλοντες κοπάριον ἢ μηλωτίδα) through its orifice, we cut the skin over it at one incision ' (VII. lxxviii).

Illustrations of two ear probes are given. What I regard as the type is seen in Pl. XV, fig. 5, which shows an instrument from the Roman Hospital at Baden. Typical specimens are not by any means common. Pl. XV, fig. 2 shows another variety from my own collection.

Screw Probes.

On probes for wrapping round with wool we frequently raise a screw thread to enable the wool to adhere better. This useful contrivance was also known to the ancients. I give a figure of one in my possession. It was found in the Roman Camp at Sandy (Pl. XXI, fig. 5). It measures 9·7 cm. in length and is 1·5 mm. thick. The screwed portion occupies 7 mm. of one end. The other end is plain. The little instrument is well adapted for treating small cavities, such as an ear or a carious tooth by wrapping round the screw portion with wool and dipping in medicaments.

Ear specillum for wounds.

Greek, τραυματικὴ μήλη ; Latin, specillum vulnerarium.

There was a special variety of ear specillum which was adapted for wounds. Paul (VI. lxxxviii) says:

'Stones and other missiles from slings may be removed by levers or the scoop of an ear probe adapted for wounds' (κυαθίσκου τραυματικῆς μηλωτίδος).

This was probably an instrument on the same principle as the ear probe, i. e. a combined probe and scoop, but on a larger scale. Possibly it may have had a slight olivary enlargement. That it was large we learn from Galen's

Lexicon, where μήλην ἰσχυράν is stated to mean τὴν τραυματικὴν μήλην. It will easily be seen that the *specillum vulnerarium* has considerable affinity with the other class of spoon probes which I constituted, viz. the class of cyathiscomeles—for these had a scoop at one end—and this being specially intended for wounds most likely had a certain amount of olivary enlargement at its tip, but smaller than the olive of a cyathiscomele, which was too large for ordinary wounds. The typical ear specilla and the typical cyathiscomeles both form well defined groups, but between these innumerable gradations occur among the specimens extant. For practical purposes it is convenient to class all these intermediate forms as *specilla vulneraria*.

Handled Needles.

In the find of the oculist Severus were no less than nine handles for needles. Of these, six were merely cylinders of bronze, expanded slightly at one end and perforated at the other with a small hole for a needle. They were from 72 to 40 mm. long and 7 to 5 mm. in diameter. Two were hexagonal, four were round (Pl. XXI, figs. 2, 4, Pl. XVI, figs. 3, 4, 5, 6). Two others had the same holes for needles at one end, but at the other they were pierced with a slot, 10 mm. deep, for the insertion of a knife blade. One was 60 × 7 mm., the other 53 × 5 mm. (Pl. II, figs. 1, 2). Another, perforated at one end as before, carried at the other an olive-pointed probe. It was 8 cm. in length, and of this 3·5 cm. consisted of a hexagonal handle 3·5 cm. in diameter. The remainder was cylindrical, and it terminated in a probe point with a slight olivary enlargement (Pl. XVI, fig. 2). In all cases the needles had evidently been made of steel and had entirely disappeared.

We have many allusions to the use of handled needles in ophthalmic work. In describing the couching of cataract Celsus says :

Tum acus admovenda est, acuta ut foret sed non nimium tenuis (VII. vii).

'Then a needle is to be applied, sharp so as to penetrate, but not too fine.'

Sextus Platonicus (*Med. ex Animalibus*) says that cataract is depressed with a specillum.

A full description of the operation is given by Paul:

' We measure off a nucleus' breadth (ὅσον πυρηνομήλης) from the part called the iris and in the direction of the outer canthus, then mark with the olivary end of the couching needle (πυρῆνι παρακεντηρίου) the place to be perforated. If it is in the left eye, we work with the right hand, and vice versa. Bringing round the pointed end of the perforator, which is round at the tip (καὶ ἀναστρέψαντες τὴν ἀκμὴν στρογγύλην κατὰ τὸ πέρας ὑπάρχουσαν τοῦ κεντηρίου), we push it firmly through at the part which was marked out until we come to an empty space. The depth of the perforation should be as great as the distance of the cornea from the iris. Then raising the needle to the apex of the cataract (the bronze of it is plainly visible through the transparent part of the cornea) we depress the cataract to the underlying parts. After the couching of the cataract we gently extract the needle with a rotatory movement' (VI. xxi).

It will be seen from Paul's vivid description that the couching instrument consisted of a handle with a nucleus at one end, to measure off the spot at which to perforate, and a needle at the other. We saw that the outfit of the oculist Severus contained one such instrument (Pl. XVI, fig. 2). The same combination is not infrequently met with. In the Museum at Aarau there are four from the station at Vindonissa. I have one in my collection which is interesting as showing a screw thread for fitting on a cover to protect the needle (Pl. XVI, fig. 7). It was found in Bedfordshire. It reminds one very strongly of the couching needle figured by Paré. Other handled needles were used in eye work as cauteries. Of trichiasis Celsus says (VII. vii):

Si pili nati sunt qui non debuerunt, tenuis acus ferrea ad similitudinem spathae lata in ignem coniicienda est: deinde candens, sublata palpebra sic ut eius perniciosi pili in conspectum curantis veniant, sub ipsis pilorum radicibus ab angulo immittenda est ut ea tertiam partem palpebrae

transsuat; deinde iterum, tertioque usque ad alterum angulum; quo fit ut omnes pilorum radices adustae emoriantur.

Ophthalmic Probe.

Greek, ὀφθαλμικὴ μήλη.

In Hippocrates (ii. 100) we find an ophthalmic probe
mentioned.

Λεπίδος μῆλαι τρεῖς τῷ πλατεῖ καὶ ἀλήτου σητανίου κόλλης, πάντα
ταῦτα λεῖα τρίψας, καταπότια ποιήσας δίδου.

'Of squama aeris three times the full of a specillum and
[as much] of the gluten of wheat. Levigate all up fine, form
into pills and administer.'

Galen in his Lexicon explains that μῆλαι τρεῖς τῷ πλατεῖ
means τῷ κυαθίσκῳ ὀφθαλμικῆς μήλης. This is the only mention
which we have of a special ophthalmic probe with scoop.
In applying medicaments to the eye with a probe whenever
any variety of probe is mentioned it is always the ear
specillum which is named. It seems most likely that either
the ear specillum or some variety of it is referred to here.
It may have had a nucleus for applying medicaments at one
end and a scoop at the other.

Rasping Specillum.

Greek, βλεφαρόξυστον; Latin, *specillum asperatum*
(Celsus).

A special burred specillum, for curetting the granular lids
so common as a result of the ophthalmia which is endemic
in most Eastern countries, and which was rampant in
ancient Greece and Rome, is described by Celsus and also
by Paul. Celsus says:

In hoc genere valetudinis quidam crassas durasque palpe-
bras et ficulneo folio, et asperato specillo, et interdum scalpello
eradunt, versasque quotidie medicamentis suffricant (VI. vi).

Paul says:

'But if the granulation be hard and yield to none of these
things we must evert the eyelid, and rub it down with pumice

stone, or the shell of the cuttlefish, or fig-leaves, or the surgical instrument called blepharoxyston' (διὰ τοῦ βλεφαρο-ξύστου καλουμένου, III. xxii).

Heister (vol. i. tab. xvi. p. 591) figures the blepharoxyston as a spoon-shaped instrument burred on the convex side. There is in the Orfila Museum, Paris, an instrument of similar form.   It consists of a handle with an olivary point at one end, and at the other a plate with transverse ridges.   This agrees well enough with what we know of the classical instrument.   It was found in Herculaneum (Pl. XVI, fig. 1).

Styli and Styloid Specilla.

Greek, γράφιον, γραφεῖον, γραφίς ; Latin, stylus or stilus.

The difficulty of deciding as to whether any particular instrument is a surgical or a domestic article is often well illustrated by styloid instruments.   In the British Museum several types of instrument will be found classed among surgical instruments, and a series of exactly similar articles will be found repeated among the styli used for inscribing and erasing characters on wax tablets.   As even the writing stylus was occasionally used for surgical manipulations we are justified in looking on all styloid instruments as potentially implements of minor surgery.   The claims of any doubtful instrument to be considered as once having been one of a surgeon's tools must be decided on such grounds as the circumstances of its discovery.

Galen (xii. 865) says teeth may be extracted with the stylus (γραφείῳ ἀνάλαβε) or with the finger.

Hippocrates (i. 46) thus describes the method of extraction of the secundines :

'Place the patient on the obstetric chair and, leaving the cord uncut, place the child on two bladders filled with water and puncture each of the bladders with a stylus (γραφίῳ) so that the water may slowly flow away.'

The writing stylus, then, from the fact of its being at hand and of suitable shape was occasionally, perhaps often, used as a surgical instrument.

I give a figure of a stylus in silver, beautifully oxidized, which was found at York while making excavations there in constructing the railway (Pl. XVII, fig. 3).

Pl. XVII, fig. 6 shows an instrument which is figured by Vulpes (op. cit.) as a specillum. Personally, I think its highly ornamented form shows that it is rather a domestic article, but, as no information is available as to the surroundings among which it was found, we can only say that its shape fits it equally well either for writing or minor surgical manipulations.

Grooved Director.

Although we have no actual description of a grooved director, we have many manipulations described in which such an instrument would be used nowadays. For example, in describing the treatment of fistulae Celsus says:

In has demisso specillo ad ultimum eius caput incidi cutis debet (VII. iv).

'A director being inserted into them down to their termination the skin ought to be incised.'

It is interesting to find that we have at least one grooved director extant to prove that this instrument was known to the Romans. It is in the Section of Surgical Antiquities of the Musée de Cinquantenaire, Brussels, and it was discovered, along with several other surgical instruments, in a surgeon's case of the usual cylindrical form.

It is 15 cm. long, 2 mm. in diameter. A deep groove runs for 6 cm. from one end. The other end terminates in a small button. It is of silver, as also were the other contents of the case. It is possible that grooved specilla may have been in quite common use, but may have been made of wood or tin, and have therefore not survived; because we learn from Galen's Manual of Dissection that probes which were used as directors in dissecting work were generally of wood, such as boxwood, so that they might not chip the scalpel (ii. 711).

Surgical Needle (three cornered).

Before discussing the eyed probes it will be well to clear the way by disposing of the needles, and of these, as the most easily defined class, it will be best to take the surgical needles first. We have innumerable references to the surgical needle though we have no actual description of it. There must have been many different sizes of it, for the manipulations vary greatly in magnitude. I shall content myself with giving two quotations describing respectively one of the largest and one of the smallest of these. Both passages are from Celsus. He thus describes the operation of suturing the abdominal parietes :

Sutura autem neque summae cutis neque interioris membranae per se satis proficit; sed utriusque: et quidem duobus linis iniicienda est, spissior quam alibi ; quia et rumpi facilius motu ventris potest, et non aeque magnis inflammationibus pars ea exposita est. Igitur in duas acus fila coniicienda, eaeque duabus manibus tenendae ; et prius interiori membranae sutura iniicienda est sic ut sinistra manus in dexteriore ora, dextra in sinisteriore a principio vulneris orsa, ab interiore parte in exteriorem acum immittat: quo fit ut ab intestinis ea pars semper acuum sit quae retusa est. Semel utraque parte traiecta, permutandae acus inter manus sunt, ut ea sit in dextra quae fuit in sinistra, ea veniat in sinistram quam dextra continuit: iterumque eodem modo per oras immittendae sunt : atque ita tertio et quarto, deincepsque permutatis inter manus acubus plaga includenda. Post haec, eadem fila eaedemque acus ad cutem transferendae similique ratione ei quoque parti sutura iniicienda; semper ab interiore parte acubus venientibus, semper inter manus traiectis : dein glutinantia iniicienda (VII. xvi).

In the next case, where Celsus describes the treatment of staphyloma of the cornea, a very small needle must have been used :

Haec fere circa oculum in angulis palpebrisque incidere consuerunt. In ipso autem oculo nonnunquam summa attolitur tunica, sive ruptis intus membranis aliquibus sive laxatis; et similis figura acino fit: unde id σταφύλωμα Graeci vocant. Curatio duplex est: altera, ad ipsas radices

per mediam transsuere acu duo lina ducente; deinde alterius
lini duo capita ex superiore parte, alterius ex inferiore
adstringere inter se; quae paulatim secando id excidunt:
altera in summa parte eius ad lenticulae magnitudinem
excidere (VII. vii).

Now for suturing tissues, and more especially tissues of
such toughness and thickness as the abdominal parietes, a
round needle is absolutely of no use. A surgical needle not only
requires to have cutting edges, as our three-cornered needles
have, but these edges need to be in good condition to work
well.   Three-cornered surgical needles were in use from very
early times.   They are fully described in the Vedas of the
Hindoos (Wise, *Hindoo System of Medicine*, p. 171).   A few
three-cornered needles of Roman origin have been found,
although they are rare.   Those which exist are of bronze.
Probably the majority were of steel, and of these none have
survived.   I give a photograph of a three-cornered needle
from my collection (Pl. XVII, fig. 4).   It is imperfect at the
point.   It measures 7·2 cm. in length, and the sides are each
2 mm. in breadth.   It is important to emphasize the fact
that only needles with cutting edges are to be looked on as
surgical, because it is not unusual to find needles, which are
round and of large calibre, described as surgical, although
they are quite unfitted for surgical work.   Such is the one
figured by Vulpes (op. cit.).

Needles of this kind are sometimes found, as this one was,
among surgical instruments.   But they are not surgical
needles in the sense that they are intended for suturing
tissues.   They are for fixing bandages.   I shall describe them
in the next section.

Round Needles and Bodkins.

Hippocrates tells us that bandages for fixing dressings
and splints on a fractured limb ought to be finished off by
stitching with a thread (iii. 55), and Celsus repeats the
advice:

Hieme saepius fascia circumire debet: aestate quoties

necesse est. Tum extrema pars eius inferioribus acu assuenda
est ; nam nodus vulnus laedit, nisi tamen longe est (V. xxvi).

⸜The round sewing needle was therefore part of the
recognized outfit of the surgeon, and numbers have been
found associated with surgical instruments. Apart from
this association with other instruments it is quite impossible
to distinguish them from domestic needles. The same may
be said of bodkins, as these too occur in surgical finds, and
are also quite indistinguishable from the domestic articles
for embroidering. Pl. XVII, fig. 2 shows a bronze needle
from Roman London. A similar one from Pompeii, now in
the Naples Museum, is given by Vulpes as a surgical needle,
owing to the fact that it was found along with surgical
instruments ; but it is evident that it is only a needle for
sewing bandages, &c.

Other types of needles and bodkins are found in bronze,
but many also are of bone and ivory. Even the latter are
quite serviceable, and in spite of their being comparatively
thick will stitch compact cloth easily. An ivory needle
from Roman London is shown in Pl. XVII, fig. 5.

Eyed Probes.

We have frequent references to eyed probes, and we also
possess a considerable number of different types. In dealing
with the dipyrene I quoted a passage to show that it
sometimes carried an eye in one of its olives. Hippocrates
refers to an eyed probe of tin. In treating of fistula he
directs us to take a rod of tin having one end pierced with
an eye (μήλην κασσιτερίνην ἐπ' ἄκρου τετρημένην), and having
put one end of a twisted piece of lint through the eye put
the probe into the fistula, get the end of the specillum,
bend it and hold the thread with the finger and withdraw
the ends. Paul quotes this passage (VI. lxxvii), but alters
the wording slightly :

'Hippocrates directs us to pass a thread consisting of five
pieces through the fistula by means of an eyed probe or
a dipyrene ' (διὰ τετρημένου κοπαρίου ἢ διπυρήνου).

Again in polypus naris (ii. 243) Hippocrates directs us to cut a sponge to the shape of a ball and tie the ball round with thread, and make it hard and of such a size as to fill the nose. To the sponge tie a thread of four pieces, each a cubit long, and make one thread of them. Put the end through a fine tin rod having an eye at the end. Push the rod bent at an acute angle into the mouth, and catch the end of the thread under the palate and pull it through, propping it with another hoof-like probe, and extract the polypus. Pl. XVII, fig. 1 shows an eyed probe from the Baden Hospital. Its shape is exactly the same as a lead probe figured by Paré for the insertion of the apolinose.

An example of a scoop at one end and an eyed probe at the other was found at Augst, and is now in the Museum at Basle (Brunner, loc. cit., Taf. I, fig. 14). It is 16 cm. long, of which the spoon, slightly defective at its tip, occupies 3 cm. About 2 cm. from its tip, which is fine, there is an elongated eye, 5 mm. in length.

Various other combinations are met with.

Ligula type of Specillum.

Greek, κυαθίσκος; Latin, *ligula*.

Ligulae are found in enormous numbers and in very great variety. They are toilet articles for extracting from tubes and boxes ointment, the various salves, balsams, and powders which entered into the mysteries of the Roman lady's toilet. The ligula is therefore not strictly speaking a surgical instrument, but as it was used by the laity, and no doubt also by physicians, for making applications to affected as well as to unaffected parts, and as it is often found associated with surgical instruments, it is advisable to bring it within the scope of this investigation. It is also convenient to do so, because some varieties approach so closely in form to the true surgical specilla that it is often difficult to decide which class to place a particular specimen in. In doubtful cases it is well to remember that the specillum is most usually a combination of two instruments

on one shaft. Brunner (loc. cit.) figures a number of ligulae
from the Swiss museums. These he names specilla oricu-
laria, although admitting that they are only domestic
articles. I have shown, however, that the specillum oricularium is a well-defined combination of scoop and probe.

Plate XVIII shows a variety of ligulae from various
sources, some simple, some combined instruments. Figs. 4,
5, 8 are most typical forms. Some of this simple type are
two feet in length. They are often overlaid with gold.
Fig. 7 shows a ligula which has so been treated. It
carries a small fork on which to poise a pellet of semi-solid
medicament.

Spoons for measuring, preparing, and pouring medicaments.

A type of spoon not uncommonly met with has a round
bowl about 2 cm. in diameter, and a handle of about
10 cm. long. Usually they are of bronze; but occasionally they are of silver, and a considerable number in bone
were found in the Roman Hospital at Baden. They are
for measuring medicaments, heating them, and removing
them from unguentaria, &c. They are often found alongside
the glass unguentaria which contained the salves. They
were also used for religious purposes.

Similar spoons with pointed handles are common in finds
of domestic articles. The sharp end is for extracting shell-
fish, &c. A larger variety of the unguent spoon has a spout
to assist in pouring the contents. This variety is rather
rare.

Pl. XIX, fig. 4 is from the British Museum. The bowl is
2·5 cm. in diameter and the handle is 15 cm. long. The
handle is round, and it has a small ringed ornamentation at
its end and one close to the bowl. The bottom has been
thinned out with heat, and there is a small perforation
visible in it. A similar spoon was found in the grave of the
Paris surgeon. Traces of medicament remain on it. This
type is probably intended for warming salves and pouring
them into the eye and other affected parts. Another variety

is seen in Pl. XIX, fig. 1. This specimen is in the Naples
Museum, and was found along with the spatula shown in
Pl. XIX, fig. 2. The handles of each are of bronze, the scoop
and spatula parts are of silver. Vulpes describes these as
a lancet for drawing blood and a spoon for collecting and
examining the same. It is impossible to regard an instrument of silver as a cutting instrument. These are for
mixing and spreading medicaments. A large spoon of
a peculiar shape from the Naples Museum is seen in Pl. XIX,
fig. 3. It is of silver. The handle, which is of ivory, is
ornamented with spiral carving, and the end bears a ram's
head. Another interesting little shovel from the same
museum is of bronze, and carries the head of Minerva
Medica on the end of the handle (Pl. XX, fig. 5). We may
here include the large double spatulae of the type shown in
Pl. XX, fig. 1, which represents a specimen from Naples.
A similar one was found in the outfit of the Paris surgeon,
and Scultetus shows precisely similar instruments in use in
his time for applying the stiffening to the bandages, &c. for
setting fractures. The Romans probably used theirs for
a similar purpose.

Tongue Depressor.

Greek, γλωσσοκάτοχος.

To open a quinsy Aetius says (II. iv. 45) :

' If the patient is adult, seat him and make him open his
mouth, and depress the tongue with a spathomele, or a
tongue depressor, and open the abscess with a probe or a
needle knife.'

In excision of the tonsil Paul (VI. xxx) bids us seat the
patient in the sun and depress the tongue with a tongue
depressor (γλωσσοκατόχῳ).

Pl. XX, fig. 6 shows one of six bronze tongue depressors,
burnished like small mirrors, from the Lépine collection
(Védrènes, *Celse*).

Uterine Sound.

The uterine sound is frequently mentioned by Hippocrates

for correcting malpositions of the uterus, and dilating and applying medicaments to the interior of the cervix. After falling into disuse in the middle ages it was reintroduced by Sir J. Y. Simpson, only to disappear once more almost entirely from sight.

I have already referred to Galen's statement that the non-pregnant os is of such a size that it will just admit an olive-pointed probe (p. 54).

Hippocrates (ii. 836) directs us to treat hysteria by dilating the cervix, first with an ointment probe and then with the finger.

Καὶ ὑπάλειπτρον καθιέναι καὶ ἀναστομοῦν καὶ τῷ γε δακτύλῳ ὡσαύτως λειοῦν.

Soranus (II. x) describes plugging for uterine haemorrhage by means of the sound :

Καὶ τρυφερὸν ἔριον ἐνί τινι τῶν εἰρημένων χυλῶν διάβροχον διὰ δακτύλου ἢ μήλης παρεντιθέσθω τῷ στόματι τῆς ὑστέρας. καὶ πολὺ μᾶλλον ἐντεῦθεν τῆς αἱμορραγίας ὑπαρχούσης.

Hippocrates (iii. 34) alludes to applying medicament to the internal os with the sound :

'Grind the pulp of colocynth, &c., and rub it up with honey and smear it on the sound (περὶ μήλην) making the consistence such that it can enter the os and always be pushed beyond until it has penetrated to the interior of the uterus. When the medicament has liquefied extract the sound, and again in the same way apply elaterium.'

If pus collect in the uterus post partum, or after abortion or from any other cause, it is good practice to pass a sound (μήλην ὑπαλειπτρίδα) into the cervix (i. 471). In another place we are directed to draw off gas in the uterus by fomenting the whole body and the uterus with vinegar and water, warmed specilla being afterwards inserted (μήλας διαπύρους ἐμβάλλοντα).

Again we find the sound applied to correct malposition of the uterus (iii. 140):

'When the semen is extruded on the third day and the

woman consequently fails to conceive, take small soft feathers and tie them together, and foment the uterus as we do the eyes. Make the feathers even at the tips and tie the ends with a very fine thread, and anoint with much rosaceum. Also place the patient on her back on a couch, and place a pillow under the loins, and, the woman's thighs being extended and separated, insert a sound and turn it to this side and that till it project.'

In all these cases there is no special instrument designated as being used for a uterine sound, only the spathomele (ὑπάλειπτρον) and the olivary probe named. With both of these we have met before. However, I have thought it of historical interest to cast these passages together. It will also clear the way for the discussion of other instruments, whose use is entirely reserved for the purpose of dilation of the cervix.

A more questionable use of the sound is referred to by many authors. During the Empire the death of the foetus was frequently procured both by abortifacients and instruments. Frequent references to the use of drugs for this purpose may be found in the lay writers such as Juvenal and Suetonius (*Domitian*), and the later medical authors do not hesitate to describe the composition of abortifacient pessaries. It will be remembered that the Hippocratic oath specially forbids this practice.

Uterine Dilators—Solid, graduated wooden.

Greek, διαστομωτρίς, μήλην τὴν διαστέλλουσαν—τὸν διαστολέα (Galen, *Lexicon*).

Besides the ordinary probes, which we have just seen that Hippocrates used occasionally for dilating the os, we have frequent mention made of a special variety of dilators which, although they are called μήλη by Hippocrates, are not, strictly speaking, probes or sounds, but a graduated set of dilators of wood, tin, or lead. They correspond, in fact, to our Hegar's dilators.

Hippocrates describes these dilators (ii. 799). The patient

is to have fumigations for five or six days till the cervix is softened. After these fumigations, dilators (προσθέτων) made of pieces of very smooth slipping pinewood are to be introduced into the cervix. There were six of these. Each was six finger breadths (4·2 in.) in length. They ended in a point, and each succeeding rod was larger than the preceding one; the largest being of the diameter and shape of the index finger, being smaller at one extremity than the other. They should be as round as possible and with no splinters. Before being introduced they were smeared with oil. First the point was gradually introduced by rotating the dilator and pushing it simultaneously till it entered for a distance of four finger breadths (2·8 in.). After the first rod was introduced it was withdrawn and replaced by a larger one. During the after treatment a leaden tube filled with mutton fat was left in the uterus at night, while through the day one of the pine dilators was used. Pl. XX, fig. 2 shows a specimen from Pompeii, which Védrènes regards as a uterine dilator. It is hollow, and is ornamented to resemble the head and body of a snake.

Metal Dilators mounted on handles of wood.

Hippocrates (i. 473) mentions a variety of dilator made of tin or lead, and hollow behind for mounting on a wooden handle:

'After douching and fumigation, dilate, and, if necessary, straighten the cervix with a dilator of tin or lead (τῇ μήλῃ τῇ κασσιτερίνῃ ἢ μολυβδαίνῃ), beginning with a fine one, and then a thicker if it be admitted, until it seems to be in proper position. Dip the dilators in some emollient. The dilators are to be made hollow behind, and fitted round rather long pieces of wood and thus used.'

This evidently refers to a portable set of dilators, each capable of fitting on a common handle, like Fritsch's, Peaslee's, or Lawson Tait's of modern times.

Bifurcated Probe.

Greek, μήλη δικροῦς, χηλή.

In treating of polypus naris Hippocrates directs us to take a sponge and tie it into a hard ball, and attach a four ply thread to it. Next to pass the end of this thread by means of an eyed probe of tin till it is caught at the back of the mouth, and drawing it out of the mouth to place a bifurcated probe under the palate, and using this as a fulcrum pull until the polypus is extracted (*De Morbis*, ii. 243 : ἔπειτα χηλὴν ὑποθεὶς ὑπὸ τὸν γαργαρεῶνα ἀντερείδων ἕλκειν ἔστ' ἂν ἐξειρύσῃς τὸν πώλυπον). In Galen's *Lexicon* we find χηλή explained as meaning a notched probe, split like a hoof at the point (μήλην δικροῦν, κατὰ τὸ ἀκρὸν ἐκτετμημένην ἐμφερῶς χηλῇ). And again under the heading δικροῦν he gives τὸ οἷον δίκρανον, ὅπερ καὶ δισχιδὲς ὀνομάζουσι τὸ δὲ αὐτὸ καὶ δηλοῖ, 'what they call cloven and also cleft.' The same word also means the notch of an arrow. In *De Morbis* (ii. 245), Hippocrates describes another method of extracting polypus with the same instrument. Taking a piece of stringy gut (χορδήν) and making a loop on it pass the end through the loop, thus making a second larger one, i. e. a noose. Pass the end of the gut through the nose into the mouth with a tin probe. Pull the loop into the nose and adjust it round the polypus with a notched probe (μήλη τῇ ἐντετμημένῃ), and when this is done pull on the gut, using the notched probe as a fulcrum.

There must have been one form of bifurcated probe with a rounded end bearing a notch like an arrow. This is the only form of cleft probe which it would be safe to use in the back of the throat in the manner described by Hippocrates. We know, however, of other forms of bifurcated probes. Celsus describes a bifurcated retractor used for the extraction of weapons buried in the flesh :

Saepius itaque ab altera parte quam ex qua venit recipienda est; praecipueque quia fere spiculis cingitur;

quae magis laniant si retrorsus quam si contra eximatur. Sed inde aperta via caro diduci debet ferramento facto ad similitudinem Graecae litterae Y; deinde, ubi apparuit mucro, si arundo inhaeret propellenda est donec ab altera parte apprehendi et extrahi possit (VII. v).

Variant readings are V and Λ. The Aldine edition has ψ. The reading I have adopted is Daremberg's; but whichever is correct matters little, as all indicate a bifurcated instrument, except the Aldine, which would indicate a three-pronged one. There are several bifurcated specilla in the British Museum (Pl. XXII). One in the Orfila Museum, Paris, of slender construction, carries a hook at the other end. It is from Herculaneum (Pl. XXI, fig. 1). A plain variety is shown in Pl. XXI, fig. 6. The specimen shown in Pl. XXI, fig. 3 is interesting as showing a possible fallacy. It has considerable affinity to the Roman netting-needle, and may not be a probe at all. The typical netting-needle has, however, blunt points, and the planes in which the forks lie are at right angles to each other.

Blunt Dissectors.

In his chapter on Angiology (or Division of the Temporal Blood Vessels) for headache and ophthalmia (VI. v). Paul mentions the use of dissectors:

'Having therefore first shaven the hairs of the temples we make an examination by palpation, applying warm fomentations or even a fillet round the neck, and mapping out the vessels with ink as they become apparent, we stretch the skin to either side with the fingers of our own left hand and those of an assistant, and make a superficial incision along the vessel. Then cutting down and retracting with hooks and exposing the vessel with dissectors (δι' ἐξυμενιστή-ρων) we must raise it up completely isolated. If it be small, having stretched it and applied torsion we may divide it through in such a way as to remove a piece of it at one stroke.'

The typical scalpel handle ends in a leaf-shaped dissector, and Celsus always describes blunt dissection as being performed with the manubriolus of the scalpel. We have, however, a few dissecting manubrioli as separate instruments not designed to carry scalpel blades. Three were found together in the grave of the surgeon of Paris. There are also two in the museum of St-Germain-en-Laye, and one in the Museum at Mainz. We may take as types two from the find of the oculist Severus in the St-Germain-en-Laye Museum (Pl. XX, figs. 3, 4). They consist of elongated leaf-shaped blades carried on hexagonal handles, and are exactly similar in appearance to a scalpel handle, except that they do not carry a slot for the insertion of a blade.

Curved Dissectors.

Greek, ὑδροκηλικὸν κοπάριον.

On the cure of hydrocele Paul (VI. lxii) says :

' When the fluid is in the tunica vaginalis we make the incision where the apex of the tunica makes its appearance, and, separating the lips of the incision with a hook, and having dissected off the fascia with the hydrocele specillum and the scalpel (ἐξυμενίσαντες τῷ τε ὑδροκηλικῷ κοπαρίῳ καὶ τῷ σμιλίῳ), we divide it through the middle with a lancet.'

Treating of the excision of varices (VI. lxxxii) he says :

' Having separated the lips of the wound with hooks, and dissected away the fascia with curved hydrocele specilla, and laid bare the vein and freed it all round ' (ὑδροκηλικοῖς ἐπικαμπέσι κοπαρίοις).

A curved dissector from the find of the oculist Severus, now in the Museum of St-Germain-en-Laye, has a neatly ornamented handle with a small hook at one end, and at the other it curves first backward and then forward to join a small leaf-shaped dissector 3 cm. long and 1 cm. in its greatest breadth (Pl. XXIII, fig. 2).

Sharp Hooks.

Greek, ἄγκιστρον, ἀγκυρομήλη ; Latin, *hamus, hamulus acutus.*

Hooks blunt and sharp are frequently mentioned in both

Greek and Latin literature, and served the same purposes as we use them for; the blunt for dissecting and raising blood-vessels like the modern aneurism needle, the sharp for seizing and raising small pieces of tissue for excision, and for fixing and retracting the edges of wounds. We are fortunate also in possessing many fine specimens of both sharp and blunt hooks in museums, &c. In the Naples Museum alone there are upwards of forty examples of hooks. Of pterygium Celsus says :

Tum idem medicus hamulum acutum, paulum mucrone intus recurvato, subiicere extremo ungui debet eumque infigere ; atque eam quoque palpebram tradere alteri ; ipse, hamulo apprehenso, levare unguem eumque acu traiicere linum trahente (VII. vii).

Aetius also mentions this use of the sharp hook :

'And, transfixing the pterygium with a hook (καὶ ἀγκίστρῳ καταπείροντες περὶ τὰ μέσα τὸ πτερύγιον), we gently make traction on it ' (*Tet.* II. iii. 60).

Paul also says :

' Seizing the pterygium with a hook with a small curve, (ἀγκίστρῳ μικροκαμπεῖ ἀναδειξάμενοι) we stretch it ' (VI. xviii).

The method of excision of the tonsil described by Celsus, Aetius, and Paul is to bring the tonsil into view by dragging on it with a sharp hook and then amputating it. Thus Paul says :

' Wherefore seating the person in the light of the sun, and, directing him to open his mouth, while one assistant holds his head and another presses down the tongue to the lower jaw with a tongue depressor we take a hook (ἄγκιστρον) and transfix the tonsil with it and draw it outwards as much as we can without drawing the capsule along with it, and then we cut it out by the root with the tonsil knife suited to that hand ' (VI. xxx).

In contraction of the vulva, Paul says :

' Having transfixed the connecting body, whether flesh or membrane, with hooks, we stretch it and divide it with the fistula knife ' (VI. lxxii).

PROBES   87

Similarly Celsus (VII. xxviii) says:

At si caro increvit, necessaria est recta linea patefacere;
tum ab ora, vel vulsella vel hamo apprehensa, tamquam
habenulam excidere.

In dissection, many of the manipulations which we perform
with the dissecting forceps were performed by the ancients
with sharp hooks. Pl. XXIV, figs. 1–5 represent specimens
from various sources; some simple, others combined with
another implement.

Blunt Hooks.

Greek, τυφλάγκιστρον; Latin, *hamus retusus.*

Aetius (*Tet.* III. i. 13) says:

'Whatever adhesions there are of the lower border of the
lids to the tunics of the eye, we must put them on the
stretch with a blunt hook (τυφλαγκίστρῳ) and with a pterygotome free the adhesion.'

In Aetius (*Tet.* II. iii) we see the blunt hook used in the
same way as we use an aneurism needle, except that the
ligature is not introduced with it, but with another needle.
He says we transfix the lips of the incisions with two hooks
and gradually dissecting with the scalpel we free the vessel
from the underlying fascia. Then with a blunt hook
(τυφλάγκιστρον) placed under the vessel we raise it up from
the depth, and beneath it when raised we place a two
ply thread by means of a needle, and doubly tie and cut
between.

Paul says:

'Exposing the vessel with dissectors we must raise it up
when it is separated all round. If it be small, having
stretched and twisted it with a blunt hook, we may divide
it through in such a way as to remove part of it. But if it
be large we must apply a double ligature under it with
a needle, either a piece of raw flax or some other strong
thing' (VI. v).

The 'eyed hook' is mentioned by Galen in describing the
dissection of the spinal cord:

᾽Ενδέχεται δὲ καὶ χωρὶς βελόνης ἀγκίστρῳ διατρήτῳ γενέσθαι

τὴν ἐγχείρησιν, ὡς ἐπὶ τῶν περὶ τὰς καρωτίδας ἀρτηρίας νεύρων εἴωθε ποιεῖσθαι (ii. 669).

'It is advisable that the manipulation be performed not with a needle but with an eyed hook, as is usually done in the case of the tendons in the neighbourhood of the carotid arteries.'

A small variety of the blunt hook is mentioned by Celsus, Galen, and Paul.

Of the extraction of foreign bodies from the ear Celsus says :

Sin aliquid exanime est, specillo oriculario protrahendum est, aut hamulo retuso paulum recurvato (VI. vii).

Paul says that if stones of fruits, &c. fall into the ear they must be extracted with an ear scoop, a hook, or a forceps.

Both types of blunt hook·are represented by extant specimens ; see Pl. XXIII, figs. 3, 4. These remind us of our aneurism needles, and it is interesting to note that Galen (*ut supra*) speaks of an 'eyed hook'. The instruments shown in Pl. XXIII, figs. 2, 4 we might look on either as curved retractors or dissectors as they are half sharp. Pl. XXV, fig. 2 shows a hook of crotchet-hook type combined with a scoop. It is from Herculaneum.

The Strigil.

Greek, ξύστρα. Latin, *strigil*.

It seems to have been a common method of applying remedies to the auditory canal to warm them in a strigil and pour them in with it. Galen frequently mentions this. In *Med. Sec. Loc.* (xii. 622) he says :

Having warmed the fat of a squirrel in a strigil, instil it.

Celsus (VI. vii. 1) says :

In aurem vero infundere aliquod alimentum oportet quod semper ante tepefieri convenit; commodissimeque per strigilem instillatur.

Marcellus (IX. 1) says :

Conteres et in strigili calefacies, et infundes, et lana occludes aurem.

Scribonius Largus (xxxix) says :

Ad auriculae dolorem et tumorem sine ulcere prodest herbae urceolaris aut cucurbitae ramentorum sucus tepens per strigilem in foramen auris dolentis infusus.

The strigil varied much in size and shape. A common form was a sickle-shaped instrument, the circular part being hollow and semicircular on section, and admirably adapted for warming and pouring oil and other medicaments into the ear as above described. Pl. XXV, fig. 1 shows a small strigil from my collection.

Spoon for applying astringent liquids to the uvula.

Greek, σταφυλεπάρτης.

In his description of the medical treatment of diseases of the mouth Paul (III. xxvi) says :

' When the uvula is inflamed we must use the gargles recommended for inflammation of the tonsils, and those of a moderately astringent nature, such as the juice of pomegranate, applied by means of a spoon or the instrument called the "uvula medicator" ' (σταφυλεπάρτου).

It is evident that it is quite a different instrument from the staphylocaustus (*q. v.*), which we are specially told had more than one hollow and was a grasping instrument like a forceps. The present instrument is for applying liquids, and was apparently of the form of a spoon. Fabricius describes and figures such an instrument. It is a small round spoon with a long handle.

CHAPTER V

FORCEPS

Epilation Forceps.

Greek, τριχολαβίς, τριχολάβιον (=τριχολαβίδιον); Latin, *vulsella*.

The removal of the hair from the face for cosmetic purposes is a custom which has come down to us from prehistoric times, and seems to have been very prevalent among all primitive races. In the bronze age the method by which this was accomplished seems to have been to fix the hairs with a broad jawed forceps and cut them off close to the skin by means of a knife or 'razor'. Thus did primitive men 'shave', and very often in early bronze age graves in Scandinavia and in the Swiss lake-dwelling excavations these forceps and razors are found together. No doubt also epilation proper was practised occasionally, but the majority of the prehistoric forceps are not for epilation but for fixing the hairs to allow the knife to divide them close to the skin. At a later time, with the more common use of steel, the Greeks and Romans shaved as we do, and epilation proper was practised for removing superfluous hairs from the face and also to remove trichiasis. Aristophanes, a contemporary of Hippocrates (Ran. 516, Lys. 89, 151), Persius (iv. 37) and Juvenal (vii. 114) refer to the depilation of the pubes as being common among certain classes, and the early Christian Fathers deplore the practice. See also the remarks of Suetonius on the conduct of Domitian (xxii). Prosper Alpinus, who visited Egypt in the sixteenth century and wrote an interesting book on the state of medicine in that country, found the custom still prevalent among the Egyptian women, and thus explains the object with which it was practised (*Medicina Aegyptiorum*, cap. III. xv):

A pulveribus, qui Aegyptiis fere toto anno ventorum terraeque siccitatis occasione perpetuo familiares existunt, atque ab assiduis sudoribus quibus coeli calore omnia corpora continue abundant, illuvieque quadam immunda redduntur, atque foetentia, ex quo pleraque ipsorum et foetere et pediculis abundare solent. Balneis omnes hi populi utuntur familiarissime pro corporum abstersione, maximeque mulieres, quibus curae magis est corpora ipsarum pulchriora facere ipsorum, illuviem et foetorem corrigentes, ut cariores sint suis viris. Eae etenim saepissime corpora in iis lavant, et mundant ab illuvie, perlotaque variis ornant odoribus ut recte unguentis oleant. Ac veluti Italae mulieres atque aliarum multarum etiam nationum ad capillorum facieique omne cultum adhibent studium, ita Aegyptiae capillorum cultum negligunt ex consuetudine omnes capillos in bursam serico panno paratam concludentes, ac ad pudendorum abditarumque corporis partium ornatum omnem diligentiam adhibent. Pudendis igitur tota cura in balneis ab iis adhibetur. Ea siquidem in primis lavant, pilisque nudant, locaque pudendorum perpetuo glabra gestant, turpeque ibi est mulierum pilis obsitam vulvam habere. Demum lotas eas partes glabrasque effectas variis unguentis etiam exornant.

The custom survived in France and Italy in the sixteenth century.

Epilation as a purely surgical operation was frequently necessary for the trichiasis consequent on the granular ophthalmia which was so common among the Romans. Paul (VI. xiii) says:

' Turn the eyelid outwards and, with an epilation forceps (τριχολαβίῳ) dragging out the offending hairs, either one, or two, or three or whatever number there are. Then apply a heated olivary probe or an aural probe or some such slender instrument to the place from whence the hair or hairs have been removed.'

The numbers of toilet epilation forceps which have been found are enormous. Moreover, forceps of exactly similar form were in use in every household as accessories of the lamp for raising and snuffing the wick, and artisans used them also for the finer manipulations of their crafts ; so that by far the largest number of forceps of this type are not surgical instruments, but household implements. However, we have plenty of specimens from purely surgical finds.

Of the surgical instruments all forms agree in having no teeth. The simplest form consists of a strip of metal bent on itself straight as in Pl. XXVI, fig. 3, or with the jaws turned inwards, as in Pl. XXVI, fig. 5. These are often pocket forceps. A 'pocket-companion', consisting of a toilet forceps, an ear-pick and a nail-cleaner, such as is seen in Pl. XXVI, fig. 4, is a common object in museums, such as the Guildhall Museum, where this object is. A variety of epilation forceps with rounded legs is seen in Pl. XXVI, fig. 2. Several of these have been obtained from purely surgical finds. Others are formed by sawing a bar of bronze up its centre, as in the specimen shown in Pl. XXVI, fig. 1, which is 13 cm. 4 mm. long, and with jaws 10 mm. broad. It is from the Naples Museum.

This is the form most typical of the surgical epilation forceps. Several of this type were found in the grave of the oculist Gaius F. Severus at Rheims (Pl. XXVI, fig. 6). They are very large powerful instruments, from 15 to 16 cm. long, and with jaws 7 to 8 mm. in breadth (Deneffe, *Oc. du 3ᵉ siècle*, ii. 1–8). This form was no doubt used as a dissecting forceps or tumour vulsellum as well as for epilation, but the typical tumour forceps was toothed, and it is convenient to classify all those of the untoothed type as epilation forceps.

Other epilation forceps, which are however more likely to be toilet articles, have the jaws of extreme breadth, as in Pl. XXVII, fig. 3 from the Mainz Museum. It has a sliding catch. They are evidently intended to remove a considerable number of hairs at once, or to fix them while they were cut with razor or shears.

It is certain, however, that in addition to these broader

forceps a variety with quite narrow blades was used, as
Paul (VI. xxiv) tells us that stones, &c. may be removed
from the ear with epilation forceps (τριχολαβίῳ), and again
in fracture of the nose Paul (VI. xxiv) says that splinters of
detached bone are to be removed with these forceps. We
have several forceps of this type. There are in the Naples
Museum three, one from Pompeii, two from Herculaneum
(Deneffe). One from my own collection is shown in
Pl. XXVI, fig. 2. The points are narrow and rounded.

A very interesting form is seen in Pl. XXVII, fig. 4,
which shows a forceps in the Thorwaldsen Museum, Copenhagen. It is 12 cm. long, of which 6 cm. of the upper end
are solid and round. The remainder of the length is
occupied by the blades of the forceps, each 5 mm. broad,
except for 12 mm. at the extremity, where it expands into
a leaf-shaped portion, 10 mm. broad in its broader part.
These leaf-shaped expansions oppose each other accurately,
and on the narrow part of the blade above them there
slides a rectangular catch which serves to clamp the blades
and fix them like the jaws of a vice.

The surgical epilation forceps is, as we have seen, usually
a simple instrument. Occasionally we meet with a forceps
combined with some other instrument. These are, as a rule,
toilet articles. A pocket ear-scoop and epilation forceps
combined was found in Paris. Precisely similar articles of
steel may be bought in chemists' shops to-day. Another
has a small unguent spatula combined with a forceps, while
others carry olivary probes. There are several of these in
the St-Germain-en-Laye Museum (Pl. XXVII, figs. 5, 2).
One from Melos, in the Athens Museum, has a porte-
caustique.

Polypus Forceps.

Greek, πολυποξύστης.

Galen (*Med. Sec. Loc.* xii. 685) alludes to the method of
extraction of polypus from the nose by means of a forceps
(ἔπειτα λαβιδίῳ ἐξαίρει), and from what Paul says it would

seem that there was a special polypus instrument, consisting of a forceps at one end and a rugine at the other. After describing extraction by means of a knife and scoop he says:

'If, however, any part of the tumour be left behind, we take another polypus eradicator (ἕτερον πολυποξύστην), and with the end of it (ἐπάκμον αὐτοῦ ξυστηρίου) bring away what remains, by stretching, twisting, and scraping it strongly.'

Ξυστήριον means a small rugine, but stretching and twisting can only be done with a forceps. Rare as the combination of an antique forceps with another instrument is, we have one example of the combination of a rugine and a forceps, and, as it is admirably adapted for the extraction of nasal polypus, I think we are quite justified in considering it to be the instrument indicated by Paul. This instrument was found in the grave of the Paris surgeon. It is elegantly formed and is of one piece of bronze sawn down the middle. The upper part is surmounted by a rugine strongly curved, pointed at the tip and cutting on one edge. The rugine measures 3 cm. in length, and 5 mm. in breadth (Deneffe, *Tr. d'un Chir.*, pl. v, fig. 1) (Pl. XXVII, fig. 1).

Tumour Vulsellum (Myzon).

Greek, μύδιον, μύγδιον, σαρκολαβίς, σαρκολάβος; Latin, *myzon, sarcolabon, vulsella.*

The form vulsellum has got so well established by usage in modern medical writings that it would seem pedantic to write 'vulsella forceps', but so far as I am aware it is not a form which has any classical authority. The classical usage is *vulsella, -ae,* feminine. I shall follow custom and use the modern term when using it as an English word.

The myzon, or tumour forceps, was a toothed instrument of the dissecting forceps type. Ducange says it takes its name from the shells which are called μυτίλοι, vulgo μύδια (mussels). It was used whenever it was desired to make

traction on any object—such as a tumour—to excise it, or to
raise and fix a piece of skin. Aetius (xvi. 106) says:

Μυδίῳ πλατυστόμῳ συλλαβὼν τὴν νύμφην διὰ τῆς εὐωνύμου χειρὸς
ἀποτεινέτω τῇ δὲ δεξιᾷ ἀποτεμνέτω παρὰ τοὺς ὀδόντας τοῦ μυδίου.

'Seizing the clitoris with a broad jawed vulsellum in the
left hand, put it on the stretch, and with the right cut it
off close to the teeth of the instrument.'

Paul gives pretty much the same instructions (VI. lxx):

Μυδίῳ κατασχόντες τὸ περιττὸν τῆς νύμφης ἐκτέμνομεν σμίλῃ.

'Seizing the hypertrophied portion of the clitoris with
a vulsellum, excise it with a scalpel.'

Aetius (xvi. 107) also says:

῞Ωσπερ οὖν ἐπὶ τῆς νύμφης προείρηται σχηματίζειν χρὴ τὴν
γυναῖκα καὶ μυδίῳ ἀποτείνειν τὴν ὑπεροχὴν καὶ τῷ πολυπικῷ σπαθίῳ
ἐκβάσεως ὅλον τὸ περιττὸν ἀφαιρεῖν.

Cf. also Paul, VI. lxxi and again Aetius (iv. ii. 3).

Again Aetius says:

'If there is a large and malignant excrescence in the
angle of the orbit, the enlarged part must be seized with
vulsella (μυδίῳ) and cut off' (vi. 74).

In the corresponding passage in Paul (VI. xvii) another
name for the vulsellum is used, viz. σαρκολάβος:—'granuloma
of the inner canthus we seize with vulsella and excise'
(σαρκολάβῳ). In treating of epulis he again uses the same
term: 'Epulis we seize with vulsella and excise' (σαρκολάβῳ).

In Moschion (II. xxx), in the chapter 'De Haemorrhoidi-
bus quae in matrice nascuntur', we find a Latin transliteration of the two terms μύδιον and σαρκολάβος side by side:

Myzo vel sarcolabo haemorrhoides teneantur ita ut in
aliquantum extensas scalpello prius radices earum scarifes,
et in aliquantum artifex sarcolabo convertat.

Here, in all probability, Soranus, from whom Moschion
is copying, has simply used μύδιον, and the added 'vel sarcolabo' is simply a gloss, for the terms μύδιον and σαρκολάβος
are synonymous. However this part of Soranus is lost.

Extant specimens of the vulsellum are common. A simple variety is formed by folding a plate of bronze on itself, as in Pl. XXVIII, fig. 1, which shows a specimen in the British Museum. The jaws are finely toothed.

More usually the myzon is formed by sawing a plate of bronze partly along its midline as in Pl. XXIX, fig. 2, which is taken from the find of the oculist Severus.

An interesting variation is seen in the specimen shown in Pl. XXVIII, fig. 3 which is from my own collection. The line of junction of the jaws instead of being in the median plane is sloping. The object of this arrangement is not quite clear. A small variety of the vulsellum is referred to by Aetius :

'Epulis we seize with a small vulsellum and excise with a small scalpel' (ἡ ἐπουλὶς μυδιοσκέλλῳ ἀποταθεῖσα ἐκτεμνέσθω σμιλαρίῳ στενῷ, vii. 24, 25).

We have one or two of these instruments. They remind one of fixation forceps. I illustrate one in Pl. XXIX, fig. 3. It is from the Mainz Museum. There are four similar ones in the Frankfort Historical Museum. The specimen shown in Pl. XXVIII, fig. 2, from the Naples Museum, is interesting as being stamped with the name of the maker, Acachcolus.

We have now to consider an interesting variation produced by extending the extremity of the blade to one side so as to increase the width of the blade (coudée type). This is a rare type.

Pl. XXIX, fig. 1 represents one of two from the find of the surgeon of Paris. It is 17 cm. long, and the legs of the forceps are 8 mm. wide. The jaws debouch to one side at an obtuse angle for a distance of 2 cm. and end in a fairly sharp point. The jaw is thus increased to 2 cm. in breadth. They are finely toothed. They are concave internally and convex externally. The other forceps was 14.5 cm. long and 8 mm. wide. The Museum at Naples has a forceps of this type, but having a sliding ring to fix the jaws after they have been applied (Pl. XXIX, fig. 4).

This angled type of forceps may be the one referred to by Paul in his description of the plastic operation on the eyelid for trichiasis (VI. viii), when he directs us to raise the redundant skin of the lid with a fixation forceps and cut it off with a scalpel (βλεφαροκατόχῳ μυδίῳ, τοῦτ᾽ ἔστι πρὸς τὴν περιφέρειαν τοῦ βλεφάρου ἐσχατισμένῳ ἀνατείναντες τὸ περιττὸν δέρμα, σμιλίῳ ἀποκόπτουσι). It may be noted that this coudée type of forceps has considerable affinity with the type of forceps presently to be described for strangling haemorrhoids and the relaxed uvula, the only essential difference being that the blades are not crossed here.

Uvula Forceps.

Greek, σταφυλάγρα.

In Aetius (II. iv. 12) we have an interesting description of the amputation of the uvula by first crushing it in a forceps so as to prevent haemorrhage and then cutting it off:

'Then inserting a vulsellum and making traction on it, the uvula crusher (τὴν σταφυλάγραν) is fitted on about the middle of the uvula or a little below it, and then it is pulled and twisted (by the vulsellum). By the torsion it becomes lifeless and, as it were, snared off; it curls up, becomes livid and comes off without much effusion of blood. Wherefore it is well to wait some time and hold it till the patient can stand it no longer, and then cut it off—the cut being made close to the vulsellum but nearer the tip than to it.'

The σταφυλάγρα therefore corresponds in its action to a pile-crusher. This instrument I believe to be represented by the type of forceps shown in Pl. XXX, fig. 1. It is in the British Museum. The two branches of the forceps cross like scissor blades, and at their ends the jaws are formed in such a way as to project forwards and enclose a cavity 1 cm. deep and 18 mm. long. Over all the forceps is 18 cm. long. The jaws are finely toothed. There is in the same museum another instrument similar in all respects except that it is 1 cm. shorter, and that in each blade, which is 16 mm. long (Pl. XXX, fig. 2), there is a small hole near the proximal end. A posterior view of a similar instrument is seen in

Pl. XXXI, fig. 1. It is from the find of the surgeon of Paris. A similar specimen is in the Mainz Museum.

Pl. XXXII, fig. 3 shows a smaller specimen from the Naples Museum. It is 11 cm. in length. A large powerful variety with a different arrangement of the handles is seen in Pl. XXXI, fig. 2 from a specimen in the Antiquarian Museum at Basle. It is 20 cm. long.

A forceps which I take to be a staphylagra occurs on the coins of Atrax in Thessaly (*circa* 400 B. C.). The forceps stands alongside a bleeding cup.

The object of the holes in several of the specimens is to permit the insertion of a cord to bind the jaws firmly together, and thus keep up the strangulation of the part for some time, as Aetius directs. The application of a ligature in this way would, of course, not be possible while the instrument was applied to the uvula, but the following passage from Leonidas (Paul, vi. 79) shows that the uvula crusher was also used to clamp piles in the same way :

'Having seized the haemorrhoids and held them there for some time with the uvula crusher (σταφυλάγρᾳ) he cuts them off with a scalpel.'

In such a case the application of a cord to clamp the jaws together would be a distinct convenience. The short variety is more suitable for external operations, as for haemorrhoids ; the long variety for manipulations in the throat.

Hippocrates mentions the uvula crusher as one of the instruments necessary for the outfit of the physician (i. 63).

Forceps for applying Caustic to Uvula.

Greek, σταφυλοκαύστης.

A remarkable variety of forceps, of which there is only one extant specimen (which is in the Vienna Museum) is shown in Pl. XXXII, fig. 2. It is formed of two branches which cross and are fixed by a rivet near the middle of the instrument. The jaws are 3·5 cm. long, concave internally, and fit accurately together, enclosing an oval cavity 1 cm. in diameter. This forceps is, I believe, the one which Paul describes as used for destroying the uvula with caustic. He says (VI. xxi) that if from timidity the patient decline excision of the uvula, we are to take the caustic used for operations on the eyelids, or some such caustic, and fill with it the hollows of the caustic holder for the uvula (τοῦ σταφυλοκαύστου τὰς κοιλότητας), and directing the patient to gape wide, and getting the tongue pressed down with a tongue depressor, we open the instrument sufficiently and grasp with it as much of the uvula as we cut off in the other operation. The medicament must neither be of too liquid consistence, lest it run down from the uvula and burn the adjoining parts, nor very hard, that it may quickly act on the uvula. And if from one application the uvula becomes black this will be sufficient, but if not, we must use it again. In VI. lxxix he says that some, filling the hollows of the staphylocaustes (τὰς κοιλίας σταφυλοκαύστου) with caustic, burn off haemorrhoids in the same way as they do the uvula. An interesting use of this instrument is mentioned by the same author in the chapter above referred to, while describing the method of treating haemorrhoids by the ligature :

'By means of the forceps for applying caustic to haemorrhoids, or the forceps for applying caustic to the uvula (τῷ αἱμορροϊδοκαύστῃ ἢ τῷ σταφυλοκαύστῃ), we surround them close to the jaws of the instrument (πρὸς τὰ χείλη) with a five-ply thread of lint, and strangle the haemorrhoids separately with this ligature.'

It would seem then that, just as there was a long instrument for crushing the uvula and a short one for crushing haemorrhoids, there were corresponding instruments for cauterizing these parts, probably differing from each other only in the length of the handle.

The passage above quoted has given much trouble to the scribes and commentators apparently from a lack of knowledge of the instrument referred to. About a third of the

codices omit τῷ αἱμορροϊδοκαύστῃ, and Cornarius and Dale-
champs reject the words τῷ αἱμορροϊδοκαύστῃ ἢ τῷ σταφυλοκαύστῃ as superfluous and interpolated. Apparently they
were unaware that both instruments were forceps of similar
principle but different lengths, and quite suitable for
putting a haemorrhoid on the stretch. The reason why these
instruments are preferred, for this purpose, to the staphylagra is apparently that not being toothed like the latter
instrument they would be both less painful and less likely
to cause bleeding.

Pharyngeal Forceps.

Greek, ὁ ἀκανθοβόλος.

Paul (VI. xxxii) describes a forceps for removing foreign
bodies from the pharynx:

 ' Prickles, fish-bones and other substances are swallowed
in eating and stick in different places. Wherefore such
as can be seen we are to extract with the special fish-bone
forceps ' (τοῖς ἰδίως ἀκανθοβόλοις προσαγορευομένοις ἐξέλκομεν).

This is the only reference to the acanthobolus I have met
with, and it gives us no information as to the appearance of
the instrument. It is noteworthy, however, that Paul in
his chapter on the removal of spiny bodies from the pharynx
is copying Aetius, and the instrument Aetius names is an
epilation forceps. He says ' bones stick near the tonsil or back
of the pharynx and can be seen, and if a considerable part
projects out of the tonsil it can be removed with an
epilation forceps (τριχολαβίῳ)'. A forceps of the epilation
type, but angled in its length, is figured by Védrènes. It was
found in Pompeii. This forceps is eminently suitable for
pharyngeal work (Pl. XXXII, fig. 1). Albucasis figures
an acanthobolus with an up-and-down, not lateral, movement.

CHAPTER VI

Bleeding Cups.

GREEK, σικύα, κύαθος; Latin, *cucurbitula*.

The extraction of blood by means of cups has been practised from remote antiquity. The Hindoo Vedas mention it, and it is interesting to note that one of the methods was to apply a gourd with fire in it, for both the Latin *cucurbitula* and Greek σικύα signify a gourd. The usual theory as to its action was that in a diseased part there was a vicious πνεῦμα which required removal.

Celsus (II. xi) thus describes the different kinds of cups :

Cucurbitularum vero duo genera sunt; aeneum, et corneum. Aenea, altera parte patet, altera clausa est ; cornea, altera parte aeque patens, altera foramen habet exiguum In aeneam linamentum ardens coniicitur, ac sic os eius corpori aptatur, imprimiturque donec inhaereat. Cornea per se corpori imponitur ; deinde ubi ea parte qua exiguum foramen est ore spiritus adductus est, superque cera cavum id clausum est, aeque inhaerescit. Utraque non ex his tantum materiae generibus, sed etiam ex quolibet alio recte fit. Ac si cetera defecerunt, caliculus quoque, aut pultarius oris compressioris, ei rei commode aptatur. Ubi inhaesit, si concisa ante scalpello cutis est, sanguinem extrahit ; si integra est, spiritum.

'There are two kinds of cups, bronze and horn. The bronze is open at one end and closed at the other, the horn, open at one end, as in the previous case, has at the other end a small foramen. Into the bronze kind burning lint is placed, and then the mouth is fitted on and pressed until it sticks. The horn one is placed empty on the body, and then by that part where the small foramen is, the air is exhausted by the mouth, and the cavity is closed off above with wax, and it adheres in the same way as before. Either may advantageously be constructed not only of these varieties of

material but of any other substance. If other things are
not to be had a small cup or a narrow mouthed jar will
answer the purpose.   When it has fastened on, if the skin
has previously been cut with a scalpel it extracts blood ; but
if it be entire, air.'

Paul says:

'When we are about to apply the empty instrument,
having placed the limb in an erect position, we fasten
it to the side, for if we apply the light above when
lying down, the wick falling upon the skin with the
flame burns in a painful manner, and for this there is no
necessity.   It is necessary that the size of the instrument be
proportionate to the part to which it is applied, and on that
account there is great difference of cupping-instruments with
regard to the smallness and greatness of size.   Moreover
those which are made with longer necks and broader bellies
are possessed of a strong power of attraction' (VI. xli).

From Oribasius (*Med. Coll.* VII. xvi) we learn that sometimes the lips were flat (ἐπίπεδα τὰ χείλεα) and sometimes
concave (σεσιμωμένα τὰ χείλεα).   This does not, however,
mean that the border was guttered, but that the whole lip
instead of lying in one plane was arched.

From a passage in Aretaeus we learn that one reason for
the cup being bellied out above was that there was oil
floating free in the instrument, which might otherwise
escape and scald the patient.   Aretaeus says:

'Apply plenty of heat so as to warm the part as well
as attract.   The cup should be light earthenware (κεραμεοῦν
κοῦφον) and adapted to the side (ἁρμόζον τῇ πλευρᾷ), or bronze
with flat lips (πρηνῆ τὰ χείλεα) so as to comprehend the parts
affected with pain, and we are able to place inside it much
fire with oil, so that it may keep alive for a considerable
time.   We must not apply the lips closely to the skin, but
allow access to the air so that the fire may not be extin-
guished ' (*De Morb. Acut.* i. 10).

Antyllus says there are three materials of which cups are
made, glass, horn, and bronze.   He rejects the silver ones
because they heat too readily.   The bronze are the ones
most commonly used.   Glass is used where we wish to
mark the quantity of blood extracted.   Horn ones are

useful about the head, where bronze ones would be difficult to remove, and also in the case of nervous persons who dread the flame. Bronze and glass cups may be used without flame like horn ones if a hole is bored in the summit and the air sucked out, and the finger or a piece of wax is applied immediately (Oribasius, *Collect.* VII. xvi).

Aristotle in his *Poetics* discusses various tricks and arts of authors and among these he mentions the riddle of which he gives as an example: ἄνδρ' εἶδον πυρὶ χαλκὸν ἐπ' ἀνέρι κολλήσαντα 'I saw a man who had glued on a man bronze by means of fire' the reference being to a bronze cupping-vessel (see also Mayor's note to Juvenal xiv. 58). The cups mentioned by Hippocrates are also of bronze. The earliest written references are thus to bronze cups worked by fire. Ethnological research would indicate, however, that horns worked by suction represent the more primitive form.

A good number of cups have come down to us. There are fourteen in the Naples Museum. There are two prevalent or usual types, one conical, and the other flatter and more rounded. The largest cup known is in the Athens Museum. Attached to it had been a chain 20 cm. long to hang it up by. It is 16 cm. in height, and was found in a tomb at Tanagra. This cup with its chain and attachment is shown in Pl. XXXIII.

In the British Museum there is one of bronze, 4 inches high and of the elongated conical shape. It was found in Corfu (Pl. XXXIV). One in Naples of similar shape has a ring attached to its summit as the Athens specimen had (Pl. XXXV).

There are four very small cups in the museum at Mainz. These are 2·5 to 3 cm. in height and 3 to 3·5 cm. in diameter. Two of these are shown in Pl. XXXVI, figs. 1, 3.

There are ten cups of glass in the Athens museum. They are of the general shape of the Mainz cups, but vary in height from 4 cm. to 6·8 cm. and in the Scottish National Museum of Antiquities there are two cupping-horns which correspond to the description of Celsus. They were brought from Shetland, where they were in use until comparatively recent times. Prosper Alpinus, who visited Egypt in the sixteenth century and wrote a book on the state of medicine in that country, found these cupping-horns in use there, and he gives drawings of the instruments he saw (Pl. XXXVII, fig. 1). The horns used were those of young bulls, highly polished and with a small hole at the tip, by which the air was extracted by suction. To close this a small tab of parchment was taken into the mouth, and moistened and affixed by the tongue. The Egyptians also used cupping-vessels of glass, specially shaped and worked by suction. Pl. XXXVI, fig. 2 shows the shape illustrated by Prosper Alpinus. The method of using fire with cups was not known to the Egyptians at the time when Alpinus wrote (*De Med. Aegyptiorum*, ed. 1541, lib. ii. ch. xii. p. 139).

Horn cups worked by suction are spoken of in the Hindoo Vedas.

It is interesting to find that these horn cupping-vessels are still in use in some parts of Africa, and one, the property of a Hausa barber-surgeon, was presented to the Aberdeen Anatomical Museum by Sir William Macgregor (*Proc. Aberdeen Anat. Soc.* 1900–2).

An interesting form of cup is described by Hero of Alexandria (B.C. 285–222). Hero's description is quite intelligible, although it would be difficult to give an accurate translation that would be readily understood. I shall content myself with summarising his account. The figure (Pl. XXXVII, fig. 2) shows a cup of ordinary flattened form, divided into two by a diaphragm. Two tubes pass through the fundus, one passing through the diaphragm, the other not. Each of these tubes is fitted with another which is open at its inner end, but closed at its outer end and provided with a small crossbar to rotate it. Each of these sets of tubes is perforated by small openings. In the case of the short tube these are outside the cup, in the case of the long tube they are inside the cup, in the chamber shut off by the diaphragm. By rotating the pistons these openings can be placed in apposition or not at will, thus forming valves. Open valve A by placing the holes in apposition. Close valve B by turning the holes away from each other. The inner chamber of the cup is now shut off except for the small hole A. Apply the mouth to the valve A and suck the air out of the chamber. Close valve A. Apply the cup to the affected part. Open valve B and the negative pressure draws on the affected part. The advantage of this arrangement is that the affected part is not directly sucked upon by the mouth, and the instrument is therefore more pleasant for the operator to use. Bleeding cups occur on the coins of Epidaurus (300 B. C.), Atrax (400 B. C.) and Aegale (200 B. C.).

Clysters.

The ancients made frequent use of injections into the various orifices of the body. The apparatus used was a bladder or skin of an animal fixed to a tube. This form of instrument remained in use till the beginning of the nineteenth century, although the elaborate enema syringe, on the principle of the force pump, had been in use since the fifteenth century at least. The following passage from Heister (anno 1739) is interesting as showing exactly the method of its manipulation:

Pl. XXXVII, fig. 3 machinam clysteri iniiciendo adaptam designat, qua Germani ut et Batavi vulgo utuntur. Litt. AA vesicam denotant cum liquore contento; quae vero in adultis duplo vel triplo amplior quam hic indicatur esse solet, pro libra circiter, et quo D excedit, liquoris continenda; BB tubulum sive fistulam osseam ano immittendam, per quam liquor in intestina iniicitur; CC vinculum superius, quod, postquam fistula in ano est, solvitur ac removetur; DD vinculum inferius, quo vesica clauditur, ne liquor immissus elabi queat (vol. ii. p. 1117).

The rectal apparatus is called by Galen κλυστήρ, the uterine μητρεγχύτης, and the bladder injector is called καθετήρ. In x. 328 we find all these three terms used in one paragraph:

Ἐς ταῦτα μὲν γὰρ διὰ κλυστῆρος εἰς μήτραν δὲ διὰ μητρεγχυτῶν

τῶν ἐπιτηδείων τι φαρμάκων ἐνίεμεν ὥσπερ γε καὶ εἰς κύστιν διὰ τῶν εὐθυτρήτων καθετήρων.

The different varieties of injection apparatus which are specially named are as follows :

    (1) Rectal: Greek, κλυστήρ, -ῆρος; Latin, *clyster*.

    (2) Vaginal: Greek, μητρεγχύτης; Latin, *clyster*.

    (3) Uterine: Greek, μητρεγχύτης; Latin, *clyster*.

    (4) Bladder: Greek, εὐθύτρητος καθετήρ; Latin, *clyster*.

    (5) Nasal: Greek, ῥινεγχύτης; Latin, *rhinenchytes*.

    (6) Ear: Greek, ὠτεγχύτης; Latin, *oricularius clyster*.

    (7) Sinus: Greek, πυουλκός; Latin, *oricularius clyster*.

Rectal Clyster.

Early Egyptian writings refer to rectal enemas : numerous prescriptions, including several for nutrient enemas, are given.

Oribasius gives us many interesting particulars about enemas (*Collect.* VIII. xxiv). The amount necessary is less for men than for women. In any case the largest amount is three heminae (τρεῖς κότυλοι), the smallest one hemina (a small half pint). In dysentery and other cases where the parts would be easily hurt, and where a prompt evacuation was required, cannulae with the opening placed in the side were used. Cannulae with the opening in the end of the instrument were used where a large evacuation was desired to be brought down from the higher parts. To destroy ascarides, cannulae with a circle of small holes placed laterally were used.

From ch. xxxii we learn that the injection pipe varied in length also, for Oribasius says that in making injections into the rectum for affections of the bladder (e. g. to excite expulsion of urine in cases of retention), the tube (τὸ κέρας τοῦ κλυστῆρος) ought to be short.

In the case of nutrient enemas Mnesitheus says the tube ought to be extremely long, and in admitting an injection one ought to keep up compression of the empty part of the clyster because it often happens that the injection returns from the rectum unless this is done (Oribas. viii).

Hippocrates (ii. 276) mentions inflation of the rectum with air by an enema in cases of ileus. A bladder is to be attached to a tube and the air injected with this. It is then to be removed and a clyster injected.

In the excavations of the Roman Hospital at Baden there was found the tube of a clyster in bronze. It is cast in one piece of stout bronze (Pl. XXXVIII, fig. 2).

Vaginal and Intrauterine Clysters.

Greek, μητρεγχύτης.

It is difficult to separate ancient descriptions of injections into the vagina from those into the uterus, for the terms for the two parts are frequently interchangeable. It is undoubted, however, that actual intrauterine injections were made. Hippocrates (iii. 17) says :

'The end of the enema (i. e. the tube) is smooth like a sound. The tube is of silver. A perforation will be made in the side not far from the small tip of the tube (καθετήρ). There will also be other perforations, which will be placed at equal distances on each side of the tube throughout its length. The extremity of the injection tube will be solid, all the rest hollow. To the tube will be attached the bladder of a sow, which has first been well scraped. Place the milk of a mare in the bladder, having taken the precaution to close the perforations in the tube with a linen rag. The bladder is then closed with a cord and given to the woman herself, and she, when the cord shutting off the bladder has been removed, puts it inside the uterus. For she herself will know where it ought to be placed. Then you press the bladder with your hand as long as pus escapes.'

The description quoted already from Heister will help to make clear the description of the manipulation. There is in the Naples Museum (No. 78,235) an injection tube of bronze answering to the description given. It is 13 cm. long, and it has at the end a small opening, while on the side, not far from the tip, eight small holes are arranged in two superposed rings (Pl. XXXVIII, fig. 1).

There is a similar but slightly smaller instrument in the same museum.

Bladder Clyster.

Greek, εὐθύτρητος καθετήρ.

There are frequent references to injection of the bladder. Although from some passages it is clear that the injection really reached the bladder, it is probable that at other times, under the heading of 'Injection of the Bladder', only irrigation of the urethra is meant, just as sometimes by irrigation of the uterus only vaginal douching is meant. Irrigation was practised by means of a bladder fixed to the end of a catheter. Galen (x. 328), however, calls the bladder syringe εὐθύτρητος καθετήρ, which may indicate that the eye was in the tip and not in the side, as in the ordinary catheter, for a catheter with a straight bore would not reach the male bladder.

Paul (VI. lix) says:

'But since we often have occasion to wash out an ulcerated bladder, if an ear syringe be sufficient to throw in the injection it may be used, and it is to be introduced in the manner described above. But if we cannot succeed with it we must tie a skin, or the bladder of an ox, to a catheter and throw in the injection through its lumen.'

It is highly improbable that with an ear syringe the injection would have passed the triangular ligament and have actually reached the bladder in the male; but the use of the ear syringe may refer to irrigation of the female bladder, and then an ear syringe would suffice.

Blacksmith's Bellows.

Greek, φῦσα.

In cases of volvulus, Hippocrates bids us insert a purgative suppository and administer an enema. If these means are not successful:

' Insert a blacksmith's bellows (φῦσαν χαλκευτικήν) and inflate the intestine in order that you may dilate the contraction both of the colon and the intestine. Then remove it and give an enema ' (ii. 305).

Nasal Syringe.

Greek, ῥινεγχύτης; Latin, *rhinenchytes.*

A special nasal syringe with a double tube is mentioned by Aretaeus (ed. Adams, vol. ii. 459). The medicament is made into liquid form and is injected by means of a nasal pipe. The instrument consists of two pipes united together by one outlet so that we can inject by both at one time, for to inject each nostril separately is a thing which could not be borne.

Galen also mentions a nasal syringe (ῥινεγχύτης), though he does not describe it (xi. 125).

Scribonius Largus also mentions it :

Per nares ergo purgatur caput his rebus infusis per cornu quod rhinenchytes vocatur (*Compositiones,* vii).

Aspiration Syringe and Sinus Irrigator.

Greek, πυουλκός.

Galen (xi. 125) says :

'In cases of sinus he uses a tube of bronze or horn with a straight bore, or otherwise the instrument called the pus extractor (πυουλκόν), which has a wide bore. But if you inject rosaceum into the former (i. e. tube of bronze, &c.) it will not pass through the syringe (πυουλκῷ), so that in that case a pipe of wide bore is to be fixed to a sow's bladder.'

This passage shows that the pyulcus differed in principle from the syringe formed by fixing a bladder on a tube. Hero (*De Spiritalibus,* c. 57) shows that it was a syringe formed of a cylinder of metal with a well-fitting plunger.

Hero says :

'And the instrument called pyulcus works on the same principle.

'For a long tube AB is made, to which let there be fitted another CD, and let C, the end of it, be closed by a plate. At D let it have a handle EF, and let the mouth of the tube AB at A be blocked by a plate furnished with a slender syringe GH, perforated.

'When therefore we wish to draw out pus, applying the extreme mouth H of the little syringe to the place in which the pus is, by the handle we draw the tube CD outward, and the space which is in the tube being emptied something else is of necessity drawn in, and since there is no other space than the mouth of the tube the liquid at and near it must of necessity be drawn into it.

'Again when we wish to inject some liquid we put it into the tube AB and taking hold of EF and pressing in the tube CD we press out as much as we think necessary.'

Note that Hero's description does not tally with the drawings which accompany the edition of his works which we possess (Pl. XXXVIII, figs. 3, 4, 5). These show an instrument with a piston formed by a plug at the end of a rod, whereas Hero says the piston is to be formed of a second tube fitting inside the first. This is interesting, because it is much easier to get a well-fitting piston in this way than in the other ; and this principle has been reverted to in many of our best hypodermic syringes and in some of the best air pumps, such as Edwards's.

Ear Syringe.

Greek, ὠτεγχύτης, ὠτικὸς κλυστήρ; Latin, *oricularius clyster*.

The ear syringe is very frequently referred to by both Greek and Latin writers ; in fact, Celsus uses the term so often to denote a syringe for a large variety of uses that it is evident that it is almost a general term for any small syringe.

In addition to its use in washing out the ear in cases of foreign bodies, impacted cerumen, &c. he uses it to wash out the foreskin in balanitis, to syringe fistulae, to wash out the bladder through a lithotomy wound, &c.

In cases of foreign bodies in the ear he says :

Sternutamenta quoque admota id commode elidunt, aut oriculario clystere aqua vehementer intus compulsa (VI. vii).

Aetius and Paul tell us it was used to wash out the vagina, and Paul says it might be used to make injections into the bladder.   Oribasius says :

'We use flushing with an ear syringe in abscess of the

intercostal space, and in fistulas to expel first the pus with warm water, then to cleanse the cavity with melicrate' (*Collect.* viii. 24).

From a consideration of the various uses to which this instrument was put, and from the fact that it is contrasted at times (e. g. in Paul, VI. lix) with syringes formed by adding a bladder to a tube, I am of the opinion that this instrument, like the pyulcus, was a syringe of the form of a metal cylinder with a plunger like the ear syringe of to-day, and used, as the ear syringe was a few years ago, for flushing sinuses and irrigating wounds, and as a handy instrument for all general purposes of the kind. This is borne out by the fact that the ear syringe, described in detail by Albucasis (p. 157), is a cylinder of bronze or silver, wide above and narrowed to a point with a small opening in it and with a well-fitting plunger wrapped with a little cotton at one end. His figure, though quite intelligible, is too conventionalised to give any additional information.

Insufflator for Powder.

Insufflation in powder form was a common method of applying medicaments to the throat and nose. All writers mention this, but the fullest description of the tube used is given by Oribasius, who says (*Collect.* xii):

' Those things which evacuate the head we use in the following manner. A reed slender and with a straight bore, six inches in length, and of such a size that it can be placed in the nares, is taken and its cavity entirely filled with medicament. The reed may be either natural or of bronze. This being placed in the nares, we propel the medicament by blowing into the other end.'

Alexander Trallianus (IV. viii) describes the insufflation of the woolly hairs of the platanus to stop epistaxis, and Aretaeus mentions the insufflation of sternutatories (459, vol. ii), and again (408, vol. ii) he says medicines may be blown into the pharynx by a reed, or quill, or wide long tube (καλάμῳ ἢ πτίλῳ ἢ καυλῷ παχεῖ καὶ ἐπιμήκει).

A fine example of a bronze insufflator was discovered among the instruments of the surgeon of Paris. It is 15½ cm. in length, and 5 mm. in diameter. It is formed by a plate of bronze bent round and soldered. It terminates in a little elliptical shovel slightly cup-shaped, of which the transverse diameter is 3 cm. and the longitudinal 3 mm.; it had originally been overlaid with gold (Pl. XL, fig. 4).

Cannulae for draining Ascites and Empyema.

Celsus describes the cannula for draining ascites (VII. xv):

Ferramentum autem demittitur magna cura habita ne qua vena incidatur. Id tale esse debet ut fere tertiam digiti partem latitudo mucronis impleat; demittendumque ita est ut membranam quoque transeat qua caro ab interiore parte finitur; eo tum plumbea aut aenea fistula coniicienda est vel recurvatis in exteriorem partem labris vel in media circumsurgente quadam mora, ne tota intus delabi possit. Huius ea pars quae intra paulo longior esse debet quam quae extra, ut ultra interiorem membranam procedat. Per hanc effundendus humor est; atque ubi maior pars eius evocata est claudenda demisso linteolo fistula est; et in vulnere si id ustum non est relinquenda. Deinde per insequentes dies circa singulas heminas emittendum, donec nullum aquae vestigium appareat.

The following passage from Paul shows that the tip was bevelled off like a writing pen :

Χαλκοῦν καλαμίσκον ... καθίσομεν ἔχοντα τὴν ἐκτομὴν παραπλησίαν τοῖς γραφικοῖς καλάμοις.

'We introduce through the incision in the abdomen and peritoneum, a bronze cannula having a tip like that of a writing pen' (VI. 1).

Two instruments answering to the above description are to be seen in the museum on the Capitol at Rome.

Another, answering more closely to the description of Celsus, is to be seen at Naples (Pl. XXXIX, fig. 2). It consists of a bronze tube, 9 cm. in length, 7 mm. wide at one end, narrowing to 4 mm. at the other end, which is bevelled off as described by Paul. Surrounding the tube and 2·5 cm. from the bevelled tip is a ring 2·5 cm. in diameter.

A more elaborate form of the cannula for ascites is seen in another specimen, also in the Naples Museum (Pl. XXXIX, fig. 3). A tube 6·5 mm. in diameter and 39·2 cm. long, has one end rounded and closed, except for a small hole in its tip and another in the side near the first. The other end carries a circular plate 2·5 cm. in diameter. Near the middle of the tube there is a slightly raised projection as if to carry a circular disc. Inside the cannula is fixed by oxidation an obturator, which carries on its end a small handle fixed on in T-fashion. Scoutetten described this to the Royal Academy of Medicine of Paris as a trocar and cannula, but the formation of the end is not such that the instrument could have pierced its own way through. It is rather an instrument which could be inserted in an incision made by a scalpel, and which could be closed after the abstraction of a certain amount of fluid—the obturator acting as an improvement on the pledget of wool described by Celsus—but otherwise inserted like the previous example. A tube on similar principles to the ascites cannula was employed in empyema (Hippocrates, ii. 259) :

'After opening let out pus once a day. After the tenth day, when everything has been evacuated, flush with wine and tepid oil. At night let out what you have put in, and when the pus becomes thin and watery insert a hollow tin tube' (ἐντιθέναι μοτὸν κασσιτέρινον κοῖλον).

Tubes to prevent Contractions and Adhesions.

Greek, μοτὸς μολυβοῦς ; Latin, plumbea fistula.

After operations on the nose, rectum, vagina, &c. it was usual to insert a tube of lead, bronze, or tin, to prevent contraction or adhesion and also to convey medicaments.

Celsus says that after the operation for occlusion of the vagina a tube of lead is to be inserted during cicatrization :

Quumque iam ad sanitatem tendet, plumbeam fistulam medicamento cicatricem inducente illinere, eamque intus dare; supraque idem medicamentum iniicere, donec ad cicatricem plaga perveniat (VII. xxviii).

A similar tube is recommended by Celsus and Paul for insertion after operations on the rectum and vagina. Hippocrates (ii. 244) and Paul (VI. xxv) direct a leaden tube to be inserted in the nostril after the abstraction of nasal polypus.

After dilation of the cervix uteri a hollow tube was put in to keep it open. The tube was also filled with medicaments which were intended to have a beneficial effect on the interior of the uterus. The fullest description of this is given by Hippocrates (ii. 799). After describing the dilation of the womb with graduated dilators, he says:

'It is necessary to insert a leaden tube, similar in shape to the largest dilator but hollow so as to contain substances, and the width of the bore will be the same as that used for ulcers, in order that the mouth of the tent may be smooth and do no damage, and it will be prepared like the wooden dilators. When the tent has been prepared fill it with rubbed down mutton fat, and when ready extract the wooden dilator and insert the leaden one.'

This leaden dilator is referred to over and over again by Hippocrates. There are in the Naples Museum three of these metal tubes. They are of bronze. One is 18 cm. long, 14 mm. wide at one end, narrowing gradually to 6 mm. at the point (Pl. XXXIX, fig. 1).

Calamus Scriptorius.

Greek, γραφικὸς κάλαμος; Latin, calamus scriptorius.

The writing pen reed is frequently referred to as an implement of minor surgery.

Alexander Trallianus (IV. viii) says that a calamus scriptorius whose joints have been removed may be used as an insufflator. Celsus (VII. v) says that when a weapon buried in the flesh has barbs too strong to be broken with forceps they may be shielded with split writing reeds, and the weapon thus withdrawn:

Fissis scriptoriis calamis contegenda, ac, ne quid lacerent, sic evellenda sunt.

Paul says 'Some apply a tube (καλαμίσκον) round about the barbs' (VI. lxxxviii).

Celsus (III) mentions a narrow tube of this sort for drinking water through in cases of nocturnal thirst.

Paul (VI. xxiv and III. xxiii) says that foreign bodies may be sucked from the ear with a reed.

Quill.

Greek, πτίλον.

Galen (x. 1011) says that warts may be extracted by means of quills of feathers.

Paul quotes this (VI. lxxxvii):

'Some, among whom are Galen, advise us to scarify round the wart with the quill of a hard feather, such as those of old geese or of eagles, and to push it down so as to remove the wart from its roots. Others do the same with a copper or iron tube.'

Aretaeus says a quill may be used for blowing powder into the pharynx (408, vol. ii).

CHAPTER VII

CAUTERIES

Cautery.

Greek, καυτήριον, καυτήρ, καυτηρίδιον σιδήρεον; Latin, *Ferrum candens.*

The cautery was employed to an almost incredible extent in ancient times, and surgeons expended much ingenuity in devising different forms of this instrument. A considerable number of these shapes are definitely mentioned. The cautery is nearly always spoken of as made of iron. Bronze becomes too soft to act well as a cautery, so that even the earliest references to the cautery in the authentic Hippocratic writings refer to cauteries as 'the irons' (σιδήρια). It is true, of course, that in special cases bronze was used—and Priscianus recommends a cautery of gold or silver for stopping haemorrhage from the throat (*Logicus*, xxii)—but iron was the usual thing, and in spite of the enormous numbers of cauteries which must have existed only a very few have come down to us, as the iron has perished. The cautery was employed for almost every possible purpose, as a 'counter-irritant', as a haemostatic, as a bloodless knife, as a means of destroying tumours, &c.

The following passage is interesting as showing its application in two of these capacities (Aet. IV. iv. 45):

'I put the patient lying on her back, then I incise the sound part of the breast outside the cancer and burn the incision with cauteries until the eschar produced stops the flow of blood. By and by I incise again and dissect the depth of the breast and again burn the incision; and often repeat the same, both cutting and cauterizing to stop the haemorrhage, for then the danger of a rush of bleeding is avoided, and after the amputation is completed I again burn all the parts to desiccation. The first cauterization is for the sake of stopping the haemorrhage, the second for eradicating all traces of the disease.'

Cautery Knife.

Greek, ξυράφιον.

Paul on several occasions mentions the use of the cautery knife. In radical cure of hydrocele, as an alternative to the excision of the sac by the knife, he explains how it may be done with the cautery, and says, 'Afterwards, when the whole is laid bare, we stretch it with hooks and remove it with a sword-shaped cautery (μαχαιρωτῷ καυτῆρι)' (VI. lxii).

Galen, speaking of cancer, says, 'Some use heated razor blades (ξυραφίοις), at once cutting and burning' (xiv. 786).

Trident Cautery.

For forming issues over the spleen Paul (VI. xlviii) says:

'Some pick up the skin with hooks and push through it a long cautery, and repeat this three times so that there are six eschars. Marcellus, however, by using the instrument called a trident or trident-shaped cautery (τριαίνη ἢ τριαινοειδεῖ καυτηρίῳ), formed six eschars at one application.'

Vulpes describes an instrument of bronze which he considers to be a trident-shaped cautery. It was found along side an instrument which I take to be a phlebotome. If it is for the purpose described above by Paul it is unusual in being of bronze, and it must have lost a good part of its teeth.

Olivary Cautery.

Greek, πυρηνοειδὲς καυτήριον.

Malignant polypus of the nose is removed, says Paul (VI. xxv), with olivary pointed cauteries (πυρηνοειδὲς καυτή-ριον); and again, quoting Leonidas, he says empyema may be opened in the same way (VI. xliv).

The special cautery which was used for 'aegilops' (fistula lachrymalis) was probably an olivary pointed cautery, as the cautery recommended by both Scultetus and Paré for this is an olivary pointed one. Paul (VI. xxii) says, 'Some after excision of the flesh use a perforator, and make a passage for the fluid or matter to the nose, but we are content with burning alone, using the cauteries for fistula lachrymalis (αἰγιλωπικοῖς καυτηρίοις) and burning down till a lamina of bone exfoliates.'

Gamma-shaped Cautery.

Paul (VI. lxii), describing the radical cure of hernia, says :

' Wherefore having heated ten or twelve cauteries shaped like the Greek letter Γ (γαμμοειδῶν καυτήρων) and two cautery knives, we must first burn the scrotum through with the Γ-shaped ones, &c.'

Obol Cautery.

In the treatise on haemorrhoids (iii. 340) Hippocrates says :

' I order, therefore, seven or eight instruments to be prepared, a palm long, and the thickness of a thick specillum, bent towards the end and flattened on the point like a small obol ' (ὡς ἐπὶ ὀβολοῦ μικροῦ).

Lunated Cautery.

Greek, μηνοειδὲς καυτήριον.

Paul says in cases of sloughing of the prepuce we must cut it off, and if there be haemorrhage we must use lunated cauteries (μηνοειδέσι καυτηρίοις). They both stop the haemorrhage and prevent the spreading of the sore (VI. lvii).

Nail, Tile and Button Cautery.

Treating of bubonocele, Paul says (VI. lxvi):

' Make a triangular mark over the centre of it and apply to the mark nail-shaped (ἡλωτούς) cauteries heated in the fire, and afterwards burn the triangle with gamma-shaped cauteries, and afterwards level the triangle with cauteries shaped like bricks (πλινθωτοῖς) or lentils (φακωτοῖς).'

Cauteries of nail shape are also referred to by Hippocrates in the treatment of recurrent dislocation of the shoulder :

' Raise up the skin. Burn with cauteries which are not thick nor much rounded but of an elongated shape (προμήκη). For thus they pass more readily through ' (iii. 151).

Galen has a long note in explanation of this term :

Φαλακρὰ κέκληκε τὰ περιφέρειαν ἔχοντα κατὰ τὸ πέρας οἷον οἱ κατὰ τὰς μασχάλας ἔχουσι πυρίνας ἤτοι τὰ διαπύρινα καλούμενα καὶ

αἱ σπαθομήλαι, προμήκη δὲ τὰ τούτοις ἐναντίως διακείμενα προσηγό-
ρευσεν, ὧν οὐκ ἔστι περιφερὲς τὸ πέρας ἀλλ' ὀξύτεραν περ' ἐμπλήρωμα
παραπλήσιόν πως τοῖς εἰς τὰς παρακεντήσεις ἐπιτηδείοις ὀργάνοις.

' He (Hippocrates) calls φαλακρά (globose) those having a
ball at the tip, such as those for the axilla, which have
olivary points and also those which are called double olivary
probes and spathomeles. But those which are the reverse
he calls προμήκη, i. e. those which have the end not globose
but rather sharp, exactly like the instruments for para-
centesis ' (xviii. 376).

In the Naples Museum there are three tile-shaped cauteries, one of iron and two of bronze. One of the latter is
shown in Pl. XL, fig. 1.

Wedge-shaped Cautery.

Hippocrates (iii. 223) says that the oblique veins of
the head are to be burned with wedge-shaped cauteries
(σφηνίσκοισι σιδηρίοισι).

Needle Cautery.

Celsus (VII. viii) says :

At ubi aures in viro puta, perforatae sunt et offendunt,
traiicere id cavum celeriter candente acu satis est, ut leviter
eius orae exulcerentur.

Treating of trichiasis he says (VII. vii. 8):

Si pili nati sunt qui non debuerunt tenuis acus ferrea, ad
similitudinem spathae lata, in ignem coniicienda est ; deinde
candens, sublata palpebra sic ut eius perniciosi pili in conspectum curantis veniant, sub ipsis pilorum radicibus ab
angulo immittenda est, ut ea tertiam partem palpebrae transsuat ; deinde iterum, tertioque usque ad alterum angulum ;
quo fit ut omnes pilorum radices adustae emoriantur.

This indicates a needle beaten out into the shape of one
of our spuds for removing foreign bodies from the eye. The
needle handles from the find of the oculist Severus are well
adapted for this work, but are dealt with elsewhere (p. 69).

Cautery guarded by a Tube.

In the treatise on haemorrhoids (iii. 345) Hippocrates
says :

' We must make a [tubular] cautery like a writing reed

and fit it to a well-fitting iron' (καυτῆρα χρὴ ποιήσασθαι οἷον καλαμίσκον φραγμίτην, σιδήριον δὲ ἐναρμόσαι καλῶς ἁρμόζον).

Again, in the treatment of polypus of the nose, he says:

'When that occurs we must insert a tube and cauterize with three or four irons' (ὅταν οὕτως ἔχῃ, ἐνθέντα χρὴ σύριγγα καῦσαι σιδηρίοισιν ἢ τριοσὶν ἢ τέσσαρσιν) (ii. 244).

Celsus says this tube may be a calamus or a tube of pottery:

Apud quosdam tamen positum est, vel fictilem fistulam vel enodem scriptorium calamum in narem esse coniiciendum, donec sursum ad os perveniat: tum per id tenue ferramentum candens dandum esse ad ipsum os (VII. xi).

Wood dipped in boiling Oil.

Hippocrates, in diseases of the liver, says that cauterization may be performed with boxwood spindles dipped in boiling oil (πυξίνοισιν ἀτράκτοισι βάπτων ἐς ἔλαιον ζέον (ii. 482). Aetius (XII. iii) says that the root of the birthwort (aristolochia) may be used in the same way.

Ignited Fungi, &c.

In the passage in Hippocrates on cauterizing for disease of the liver, Hippocrates, as an alternative to the hot iron, says that eschars may be produced by fungi. This must mean that they were set on fire like the old moxa.

This is probably what is meant by Paul when, in treating of cauterizing over the stomach, he says (VI. xlix):

'But some do not burn with iron but with the substances called iscae. The iscae (ἴσκαι) are spongy bodies forming on oaks and walnut trees, and are mostly used among the barbarians.'

Aetius (II. iii. 91) says iscae are the medullary wood of the walnut tree.

In Hippocrates (ii. 482) the word μύκης, a fungus, is used—ἢ μύκησιν ὀκτὼ ἐσχάρας καῦσαι (or with fungi burn eight scars).

CHAPTER VIII

BONE AND TOOTH INSTRUMENTS

Raspatory.

GREEK, ξυστήρ; Latin, *scalper excisorius, scalper medicinalis.*

The raspatory or rugine consists of a blade of varying shape fixed at right angles to the shaft, and it is operated by pulling instead of by being driven forwards by striking or pushing. Although no ancient raspatory has been preserved to us we are quite familiar with the instrument, as it has been in continuous use throughout ancient and mediaeval times, and it is in use at the present day. The raspatory is the instrument upon which Hippocrates relies for eradicating fissured and contused bone in injury to the skull:

'If you cannot discover whether the bone is broken or contused, or both the one and the other, nor can see the truth of the matter, you must dissolve black ointment and fill the wound with the solution, and apply a linen rag smeared with oil, and then a poultice of maza with a bandage; and on the next day, having cleaned out the wound, scrape the bone with the raspatory (ἐπιξύσαι). And if the bone is not sound but fractured and contused, the rest of the bone will be white when scraped, but the fracture and contusion, having imbibed the preparation, will appear black, while the rest of the bone is white. And you must again scrape more deeply the bone where it appears black, and if you thus remove the contusion and cause it to disappear you may conclude that there has been a contusion of the bone to a greater or less extent, which has occasioned the fracture that has disappeared under the raspatory' (ὑπὸ τοῦ ξυστῆρος) (iii. 366).

From Galen we learn that there were different sizes and shapes of the raspatory (x. 445):

'In simple fissure reaching to the second plate narrow

raspatories are used, and they should be of different sizes to suit all cases. The affected bone being exposed *secundum artem*, first the broader ones are to be used, then the smaller down to the narrowest. The narrowest are to be used in the diploe.'

Paul refers to a small raspatory (ξυστήριον) for use as a tooth scaler (q. v.). All the mediaeval writers figure numerous shapes of raspatories—many more than we use to-day, but all on the same principle as ours.

Chisel.

Greek, ἐκκοπεύς; Latin, *scalper, scalprum planum.*

The flat chisel is referred to by Celsus in his description of the levelling of an elevation on one side of a depressed fracture of the cranium :

Ergo, si ora alteri insedit, satis est id quod eminet plano scalpro excidere ; quo sublato, iam rima hiat quantum curationi satis est (VIII. iv).

Numerous references occur in other authors. There is a fine example of a flat chisel in the Cologne Museum (Pl. XLI, fig. 2). It is all of steel, and delicately ornamented with spiral indentations. This interesting little instrument was found in the surgeon's outfit already described, and is one of the best authenticated instruments— as regards its having been the property of a surgeon—we possess. The chisel figured by Vulpes, consisting of a cylindrical bronze handle and a flat blade, is, I believe, a variety of scalpel.

We have many interesting references to the use of the chisel in bone work. It was used as an osteotome to divide the bone in distorted union :

' If the callus be of stony hardness incise the skin with a scalpel, and divide the union with chisels ' (ἐκκοπεῦσι) (Paul, VI. cix).

In the removal of supernumerary digits we are to cut away the flesh all round, and either chop the bone through with a chisel (τῷ ἐκκοπεῖ), or remove it by sawing (Paul,

VI. xliii). In using the chisel as an osteotome one chisel
was often placed behind the bone to steady it while it was
being struck by another in front. This method of applying
two chisels, which is only described by the Greek authors,
is always referred to by the phrase ἐκκοπέων ἀντιθέτων.

The following passage from Galen fully describes the
manipulation (ii. 687):

' Separate off the membranes adhering to the bone, which
being properly done, divide the bone of the rib by means
of two chisels placed in opposition to each other *secundum
artem*' (ἀντιβαλλομένων δυοῖν ἀλλήλοις ἐκκοπέων ὡς ἔθος).

The following passage from Paul shows the chisel used
for a similar purpose:

' If part of the clavicle is broken off and unconnected,
and if we find it irritating the parts, we must make
a straight incision with a scalpel and remove the broken
portion and smooth it with chisels (δι' ἐκκοπέων), taking care
that the instrument called 'meningophylax' (q. v.), or
another chisel, be put under the clavicle (μηνιγγοφύλακος ἢ
ἑτέρου ἐκκοπέως) to steady it' (VI. xciii).

The phrase δι' ἐκκοπέων ἀντιθέτων, which Paul uses in
describing the treatment of a fistula leading to carious
bone, is translated by Briau—'à l'aide de tenailles tran-
chantes'. It does seem here, and occasionally in other
passages, as if the phrase might suggest 'cutting forceps',
but we have no knowledge of such an instrument being
used by surgeons in classical times, and the passages from
Paul and Galen show that only two chisels are meant.
We may compare the passage on extraction of the foetus
in Paul (VI. lxxiv), where he directs a second hook to be
fixed on opposite the first (καὶ ἀντίθετον τούτῳ δεύτερον).

Gouge.

Greek, κυκλίσκος, κοιλισκωτὸς ἐκκοπεύς, κυκλισκωτὸς ἐκκοπεύς,
σκυλισκωτὸς ἐκκοπεύς; Latin, *scalper excisorius*.

The Greek writers frequently refer to the gouge. Celsus
never does so by any special name, although it is evident

that many of the manipulations he describes as being performed by the 'scalper', his general term for chisels of all kinds, could only be performed with gouges and not with flat chisels. The gouge was a favourite instrument of Galen's, especially in injury to the skull. With it he removed pieces of fractured bone from the skull. He also used it to groove a path for the vertical cutting instrument called the lenticular (q. v.). He calls it a 'hollow chisel' (τῶν κοίλων ἐκκοπέων οὓς καὶ κυκλίσκους ὀνομάζουσιν, x. 445).

Paul (VI. xc) says:

'And if the bone be weak, naturally, or from the fracture, we cut it out with gouges (σκυλισκωτοῖς), beginning first with the broader ones, and changing to the narrower, and then using those which are probe-like, striking gently with the mallet to prevent concussion of the head.'

The gouge is still familiar to us.

Lenticular.

Greek, φακωτός.

The lenticular of the ancients was a vertical chisel cutting on one edge and struck on the other by a hammer, while the end carried a rounded button, which being smooth did not injure the brain (Pl. XL, fig. 4). It takes its name from the lentil-like (φακωτός) shape of the button. Galen had a high appreciation of it, and gives a full description of its principle (x. 445), which is transcribed by Paul (VI. xc):

'The method of operating with a sort of incisor called lenticular is greatly praised by Galen, being performed without drilling after the part has been grooved all round with gouges.'

Wherefore he says:

'If you have once exposed the place, then applying the chisel, which has at its point a blunt (rounded), smooth, lentil-shaped knob, but which longitudinally is sharp, when you apply the flat part of the lenticular to the meninges divide the cranium by striking with the small hammer. For we have all that we require in such an operation, for the membrane, even if the operator were half asleep, could

not be wounded, being in contact only with the flat part of
the lenticular, and if it be adherent anywhere to the calvarium the flat part of the lenticular removes its adhesion
without trouble.   And behind it follows the incisor or
lenticular itself, dividing the skull, so that it is impossible
to discover another method of operating more free from
danger or more expeditious.'

The earliest illustration of the lenticular I have been able
to obtain is that given by Vidus Vidius (Pl. XL, fig. 2).
It evidently is the same instrument as that described by
Galen.

Hammer.

Greek, σφῦρα; Latin, *malleolus.*

I have already quoted passages where the hammer is
referred to as being used in cranial surgery.   Paul says :
'When you apply the flat part of the lenticular to the
meninges divide the skull by striking with a small
the hammer,' and again in using gouges, 'strike gently with
hammer (σφῦρα) to avoid concussion of the head' (VII. xc).

Paul and Celsus describe a method of extracting foreign
bodies from the ear by laying the patient on a board and
striking the under side with a mallet.   Paré mentions
a hammer made of lead, and Fabricius describes one padded
with leather, but neither of these is described by the
ancients.   There is, however, a Roman hammer of lead from
the excavation at Uriconium in the Shrewsbury Museum.

Block.

Greek, ἐπίκοπον, a butcher's block.

The ancients frequently amputated parts by placing them
on a block and striking them with a chisel.   The mediaeval
surgeons amputated parts as large as the forearm in this
way, but the Greeks all describe amputation by knife and
saw.   We have reference to the 'block' in Greek literature,
however.   In describing the plastic removal of a portion of
the scrotum Paul (VI. lxvii) says :

'Leonidas, laying the patient on his back, cuts off the
redundant portion upon a chopping block of any kind of

wood or stiff leather' (κατ' ἐπικόπου σανιδίου τινὸς ἢ σκληροῦ δέρματος).

Galen uses the same word in the eighth book of his work on Practical Anatomy—apologizing somewhat for calling the article used by anatomists and surgeons by the undignified term of butcher's block :

Χρώμενος ἐπικόπῳ, καλέσαι γὰρ οὕτως οὐδὲν χεῖρον ἔστιν ὁμοίως τοῖς ἀνατομικοῖς τε καὶ χειρουργοῖς τὸ στήριγμα τῶν ὑποβεβλημένων τῇ τομῇ τῶν σωμάτων (ii. 685).

Meningophylax.

Greek, μηνιγγοφύλαξ ; Latin, membranae custos.

The meningophylax was a small plate, which was inserted under a bone which was being cut in order to protect underlying structures. 'In cutting or sawing the bone,' says Paul (VI. lxxvii), 'when any vital parts are situated below, such as the pleura, spinal marrow, or the like, we must use the instrument called the meningophylax for protecting them (μηνιγγοφύλακα).'

Celsus thus describes it (VIII. iii) :

Factis foraminibus eodem modo media septa, sed multo circumspectius, excidenda sunt, ne forte angulus scalpri eandem membranam violet ; donec fiat aditus, per quem membranae custos immittatur ; μηνιγγοφύλακα Graeci vocant. Lamina aenea est, firma paulum resima, ab exteriore parte laevis ; quae demissa sic ut exterior pars eius cerebro proprior sit, subinde ei subiicitur quod scalpro discutiendum est ; ac si excipit eius angulum, ultra transire non patitur ; eoque et audacius, et tutius, scalprum malleolo medicus subinde ferit, donec undique excisum os eadem lamina levetur, tollique sine ulla noxa cerebri possit.

Pl. XL, fig. 3 shows a figure of the meningophylax from Vidius.

Drill.

Greek, τρύπανον ; Latin, terebra, terebella.

There are, says Celsus, two kinds of drills. The first like those used by artisans and driven by a thong, the second with a guard to prevent the instrument from sinking too deeply into the bone. The drill was used in excising a piece of the skull where the diseased portion was larger than could be comprehended by the modiolus of a trephine. The part to be removed was surrounded by perforations with the drill and the intervening spaces were divided with chisels or raspatories. Celsus says:

At si latius vitium est quam ut illo comprehendatur, terebra res agenda est. Ea foramen fit in ipso fine vitiosi ossis atque integri ; deinde alterum non ita longe, tertiumque, donec totus is locus qui excidendus est his cavis cinctus sit. Atque ibi quoque, quatenus terebra agenda sit, scobis significat. Tum excisorius scalper ab altero foramine ad alterum malleolo adactus id quod inter utrumque medium est excidit ; ac sic ambitus similis ei fit qui in angustiorem orbem modiolo imprimitur (VIII. iii).

Paul says:

'If a weapon be lodged deep in bone of considerable thickness it may be bored out with drills' (τρυπάνοις) (VI. lxxxviii).

Aretaeus (ed. Adams, p. 467) says that exposed bones are to be surrounded with perforations by means of the drill and thus reduced (τερέτρῳ χρὴ περικόπτειν τὰ γυμνά).

The boring parts of drills are not unfrequently found. The most ancient illustrations known to me of drills driven by thongs are in the work by Vidus Vidius (*Chirurgia e Graeco in Lat. Conversa*, V. Vidio. Florent. interprete c. nonn. eiusd. commentariis. Lutec. Paris., 1544).

Vidius shows three arrangements for driving these drills with thongs: the first method consists simply of a thong attached to the shaft of the drill (Pl. XLII, fig. 4); the second consists of a bow with the string of the bow wound once round the shaft (Pl. XLII, fig. 5); and the third consists of a crosspiece with a hole in the centre of it through which the shaft passes, and having strings from the end of the crosspiece to the top of the shaft (Pl. XLII, fig. 3). Primitive arrangements truly, yet all three methods of producing rotary motion are to be seen in use at the present day, and be it known that some of the most delicate boring performed by the hand of man at the present day is done with drills turned by the thong stretched across a bow.

The latest developments in mechanical devices for drilling have failed to displace thong-driven drills for boring the holes in which the wheel spindles of the best hand-made chronometers move, and the spindles themselves are turned in chucks rotated not by belts in continuous rotary motion, but in alternating motion by means of a thong stretched across a bow. A bow of cane with a strong but fine thread, one turn of which is taken round the drill, is drawn backwards and forwards and rotates the drill with marvellous rapidity and accuracy. The bows used by watchmakers average about a foot along the string. Similar drills are used by engineers in turning out small work. The form with the crosspiece may be seen in use by travelling crockery menders, who drill holes in broken pottery and clamp the pieces with rivets. A turn or two of the string is made round the shaft, and the point of the drill being adjusted on the spot to be bored the crosspiece is gently pressed down by the first and third fingers, causing the shaft to rotate. When the thong has nearly uncoiled itself the pressure is slightly removed, the momentum causes the shaft to overrun and coil the thong in the opposite direction to which it originally was. The crosspiece is again depressed and the alternating rotation goes on without intermission, and the drill bores through the pottery. The travelling crockery mender is, in the northern towns of England, not an unusual sight squatting at work on the kerb. On the continent the 'Rastelbinder' is a regular domestic institution. Not only crockery but glass is readily drilled by these means, and one who has seen the rapidity with which these drills rotate can readily understand the necessity for the advice given both by Hippocrates and Celsus to frequently remove the drill and dip it in cold water, in case sufficient heat be generated by the friction to cause subsequent exfoliation of the neighbouring bone.

The remaining method of producing rotation by means of a string fixed to the shaft can be seen in use by boatmen when clearing water out of a boat with a mop,

The mop is laid over the side of the boat.   A few turns of
a rope fixed to the shaft are made round it and the rope
being pulled the shaft rotates.   The momentum generated
causes the shaft to overrun and the rope to coil itself in
the reverse way to the original.   This is repeated till the
speed generated causes the water to fly off the mop by cen-
trifugal motion.

The fire drill of the ancient Egyptians was turned by
a bow, and it is interesting in connexion with the advice of
Hippocrates to avoid generating too much heat in drilling
the skull, and also because it helps to explain the construction
of the instruments of Vidius.   A sketch of an ancient fire
drill found by Flinders Petrie (*Ten Years Digging in Egypt*)
shows that the head of the drill was separate and the points
were also removable.

Drill with Guard.

Greek, τρύπανον ἀβάπτιστον ; Latin, *terebra abaptista.*

This is the second variety of drills described by Celsus.
It had a collar which prevented it from sinking beyond a certain depth, so that in excising a piece of bone from the skull,
which was the object for which it was used, there was little
danger of its doing injury to the brain or its membranes :

Terebrarum autem duo genera sunt ; alterum simile ei
quo fabri utuntur ; alterum capituli longioris, quod ab
acuto mucrone incipit, deinde subito latius fit ; atque iterum
ab alio principio paulo minus quam aequaliter sursum
procedit (VIII. iii).

Further on in the same passage Celsus states that they
were to be frequently removed and dipped in water lest too
great heat should be generated, so that they were evidently
driven at a rapid rate with a thong like the other drills.
They are not mentioned by Hippocrates, but Galen (x.
445) describes them :

' In order to make less chance of error they have invented
drills called abaptista (ἀβάπτιστα τρύπανα), which have a
circular border a little above the sharp point of the drill.

It is best to have several for every thickness of the calvarium ; for thicker bone longer are required, for thinner
bone shorter.'

Paul (VI. xc) says :

' But if the bone is strong it is first to be perforated with
that kind of perforators called abaptista (περιτρυπήσαντες
ἀβαπτίστοις τοῖς λεγομένοις), which have certain eminences to
prevent them sinking down to the membrane, and then
with chisels we remove the bone not whole, but in pieces.'

The illustrations of drills given from Vidius (Pl. XLII)
are really abaptista.

Saw.

Greek, πρίων, μαχαιρωτὸς πρίων (as if from μαχαιρόω) ; Latin,
serrula.

The saw is very frequently mentioned in the description
of operation on bone. Celsus (VII. xxxiii), in describing
the amputation of a gangrenous limb, says :

Dein id serrula praecidendum est, quam proxime sanae
carni etiam inhaerenti : ac tum frons ossis, quam serrula
exasperavit, laevanda est.

And Paul says that in amputating a gangrenous limb
the flesh ought to be retracted with a band lest it be torn
by the saw. Saws were also used in cranial surgery.
Hippocrates frequently mentions a saw (πρίων) in this connexion, but it is evident that he means the trephine, as he
describes its circular motion. Paul, however, makes it
quite clear that he means flat cranial saws, for he mentions
both saws and trephines in one paragraph :

Ἤδη καὶ τῶν πριόνων τε καὶ χοινικίδων χειρουργίαι, κτλ.

' The method of operating with saws and trephines is
condemned by the moderns as a bad one ' (VI. xc).

Pl. XLI, fig. 3 shows a surgical saw from the British
Museum (No. 2,328). It is of bronze, and measures 112 mm.
long, 3 cm. broad at one end, narrowing to 23 mm. at the other.
There are surgical saws of steel in the Naples Museum. Many
of the saws extant are for use as 'frame' saws. Others have
the saw portion continuous with the handle, like a knife.

Galen (xviii. 331) mentions these 'knife-shaped' saws :
'For in this way each does not become so exactly smooth
as with sword-shaped saws (μαχαιρωτῶν πριόνων).' There
is an example of this form of saw in the Guildhall Museum,
London.

Trephine.

Greek, τρύπανον, πρίων, πρίων χαρακτός, χοινικίς, ὀρθοπρίων;
Latin, *modiolus.*

The ancient trephine is referred to by Hippocrates, who
mentions a saw (πρίων and πρίων χαρακτός) having a circular
motion (iii. 374) :

'In trephining you must frequently remove the trephine,
on account of the heat in the bone, and plunge it in cold
water.   For the trephine (πρίων), being heated by the
circular motion (περιόδου) and heating and drying the bone,
burns it and makes a larger piece of bone exfoliate than
would otherwise be necessary.'

And again :

' You must saw the bone down to the meninges with
a serrated trephine (πρίονι χρὴ χαρακτῷ ἐμπρίειν), and in doing
so must take out the trephine (πρίονα), and examine with
a probe and by other means along the track of the trephine '
(πέριξ κατὰ τὴν ὁδὸν τοῦ πρίονος).

In injuries to the head in young people (iii. 371) he
mentions a small trephine (σμικρὸν τρύπανον), so that
apparently several sizes were available.   Hippocrates, we
have seen, uses the words πρίων and πρίων χαρακτός to denote
the trephine.   Galen always uses χοινικίς, but in his Lexicon
he gives two other words, viz. ὀρθοπρίονι and περητηρίῳ,
ostensibly from the works of Hippocrates:

Ὀρθοπρίονι—τῇ χοινικίδι.

περητηρίῳ—τρυπάνῳ τῷ εὐθεῖ καὶ ὀξεῖ, ἔστι γὰρ καὶ ἔτερον ἡ
χοινικίς.

These terms do not, however, occur in any extant Hippocratic writings, unless, as seems possible to me, the latter
term περητηρίῳ be a *var. lect.* for the obscure word τρυγλη-

τηρίῳ applied to τρύπανον in ii. 470 in the description of trephining a hole through a rib to drain an empyema. Galen held the trephine in little esteem. It must have been difficult to manufacture a satisfactory instrument of bronze. In x. 448 he says : 'Some people, shall I call them rather cautious or rather timid, have used trephines' (χοινικίσιν); and Paul, in a passage I have already quoted, says : 'The mode of operating with saws and trephines is condemned by moderns as a bad one.'

The term χοινικίς is derived from χοινίκη and χνόη, the nave of a wheel. The Latin term for the trephine, *modiolus*, has the same meaning. Celsus graphically describes the trephine and the method of its application. From him we learn how the ancients solved the problem of the centre-pin, which is necessary until the toothed portion has begun to bite. In modern trephines this difficulty is got over by withdrawing the pin up the centre of the shaft. In mediaeval trephines it was solved by providing two instruments, a male and a female, the male with centre-pin being used till a circular track had been cut by the toothed ring, the female without pin being then used. In the time of Celsus the centre-pin was removable, being taken out after the instrument had begun to bite. From Celsus too we learn that the trephine was driven by a thong.

Celsus and Hippocrates both remark that, as in the case of the drill, it is necessary to dip the trephine in cold water at intervals in order to cool it, lest heat sufficient to injure the surrounding bone be generated. The thong manipulated by a bow would seem to be the method most applicable to an instrument like the trephine, which has a large boring radius, as slower motion is more easily produced by this arrangement than by one consisting of a cross-piece with thongs. Celsus says:

Exciditur vero os duobus modis : si parvulum est quod laesum est, modiolo, quem χοινικίδα Graeci vocant : si spatiosius, terebris. Utriusque rationem proponam. Modiolus ferramentum concavum teres est, imis oris serratum ;

per quod medium clavus, ipse quoque interiore orbe cinctus, demittitur. Terebrarum autem duo genera sunt: alterum simile ei quo fabri utuntur: alterum capituli longioris, quod ab acuto mucrone incipit, deinde subito latius fit; atque iterum ab alio principio paulo minus quam aequaliter sursum procedit. Si vitium in angusto est quod comprehendere modiolus possit, ille potius aptatur: et si caries subest, medius clavus in foramen demittitur; si nigrities, angulo scalpri sinus exiguus fit qui clavum recipiat ut, eo insistente, circumactus modiolus delabi non possit: deinde is habena, quasi terebra convertitur. Estque quidam premendi modus, ut et foret et circumagatur; quia si leviter imprimitur parum proficit, si graviter non movetur. Neque alienum est instillare paulum rosae vel lactis, quo magis lubrico circumagatur; quod ipsum tamen, si copiosius est, aciem ferramenti hebetat. Ubi iam iter modiolo impressum est, medius clavus educitur, et ille per se agitur: deinde, quum sanitas inferioris partis scobe cognita est, modiolus removetur.

Perforator for Fistula Lachrymalis.

Greek, λεπτὸν τρύπανον.

Galen (xii. 821) says that Archigenes in cases of fistula lachrymalis perforated the nasal bone with a small drill (λεπτὸν τρύπανον), and Paul (VI. xxii) says:

Some, after excision of the flesh, use a perforator (τρύπανον) and make a passage for the fluid or matter to the nose.

Albucasis figures a drill for this purpose which he says had a triangular iron point and a conical wooden handle.

In the find of instruments of the third-century oculist Severus is a drill which Deneffe regards as intended for this purpose. It is 6 cm. in length and 7 mm. on each of its four sides. One end is pointed, the other has a slit for a knife-blade. It is beautifully damascened with silver (Pl. II, fig. 7).

Bone Lever.

Greek, μοχλίσκος, ἀναβολεύς.

Instruments for levering fractured bones into position are described in several places. Hippocrates (iii. 117) says:

'In those cases of fracture in which the bones protrude
and cannot be restored to their place, the following mode
of reduction may be practised : pieces of steel (σιδήρια) are
to be prepared like the levers (οἱ μοχλοί) which the cutters
of stone make use of, one being rather broader and the
other narrower, and there should be at least three, or even
more, so that you may use those that suit best, and then
along with extension we must use these as levers, applying
the under surface of the piece of iron to the under fragment
of bone, and the upper surface to the upper bone, and in
a word we must operate powerfully with the lever as we
would do upon a stone or a log. The pieces of steel should
be as strong as possible so that they may not bend.'

In a note to this passage Galen (xviii. 593) says:

'It is evident that the instruments described resemble
those of stone cutters, not in size but in principle. For the
instruments prepared by us for levering bone are similar in
size to those used for levering out teeth. But for levering
bones several ought to be prepared, differing from each other
in length as well as breadth and thickness at the point, by
which means they may afford their greatest effect.'

Paul (VI. cvi) gives us some additional information :

'Of whatever bones therefore we endeavour to replace
the protruded ends, we must not meddle with them when
in a state of inflammation. But on the first day before
inflammation has come on, or about the ninth day after
inflammation has gone off, we may set them with an instrument called the lever (τῷ λεγομένῳ μοχλίσκῳ). It is an
instrument of steel about seven or eight fingers' breadth in
length, of moderate thickness that it may not bend during
the operation, with its extremity sharp, broad, and somewhat curved.'

There are two bone levers in the Naples Museum, both of
bronze. Pl. XLI, fig. 1 shows one of them (No. 78,012). It is
15·5 cm. in length, and with its ends flattened, and curved,
and pointed, as described by Paul. The other instrument is
of similar shape, but is somewhat less in size. The concave
surface at one end is smooth, at the other ridged like a file.

It may be remarked, that though the similarity in form
to the instruments figured by Paré as in use in his time
for levering up depressed bones shows that these are un-

doubtedly bone levers, it is quite possible, from what Galen says, that they may also have been used for levering out teeth. The smooth end also corresponds to the description of the meningophylax, so that it is possible it may have been used in that capacity also.

Bone Forceps.

Greek, ὀστάγρα.

Galen (x. 450) says, in comminuted fracture of the skull we must make a way for the lenticular with the bone forceps (διὰ τῆς ὀστάγρας); and in depressed fracture Paul (VI. xc) says:

'If the bone is strong it is first to be perforated with the drills called abaptista and the fractured bone is to be removed in fragments, with the fingers if possible, if not, with a tooth forceps or a bone forceps' (ὀδοντάγρα ἢ ὀστάγρα).

Soranus (lxiv. p. 366) says that in impaction of the foetal cranium the head may be opened with a sharp instrument and the pieces of the skull removed with tooth or bone forceps (ὀδοντάγρας ἢ ὀστάγρας). Aetius copies this (IV. iv. 24) and so does Paul (VI. lxxiv).

An excellent specimen of the sequestrum forceps was found in the house of the physician at Pompeii, and is now in the Museum at Naples (No.78,029). It is formed of two crossed branches moving on a pivot. The handles are square, the jaws are curved, and have across the inside of them parallel grooves which oppose each other accurately (Pl. XLIII). It is classed in the catalogue as an instrument for crushing calculus of the bladder. This is, however, not a manipulation which is described by the ancients. The only case in which splitting of calculi is referred to is in Celsus, and then a chisel is used.

Varix Extractor.

An instrument, apparently a forceps, for extracting varicose veins in segments is mentioned by Galen:

'And with regard to varices in the legs, first having mapped them out on the surface with scarifications, then setting about the operation, taking hold of the skin we divide it first. Then pulling up the varix with a hook we tie it, and, doing this at all the cuts in the skin, and cutting the ends, we either remove it with a varix extractor (κιρσουλκῷ) or, taking hold of it with a doubled thread, we draw it through the channel of the varix after the manner of flaying' (xiv. 790).

Celsus (VII. xxxi) directs us to expose the vein and raise it by a blunt hook at intervals of four finger breadths, and divide the vein at one hook and pull the vein out at the next place. Galen, however, indicates that there was a special instrument for the purpose, and this can scarcely have been anything else than a forceps of some kind. The operation must have been excessively painful. Pliny (xi. 104) remarks that C. Marius was the only man who had undergone it in the upright position.

Blacksmith's Tongs.

Latin, *vulsella quali fabri utuntur.*

For replacing a protruding bone in a case of compound fracture Celsus (VIII. x) says that a forceps such as smiths use may be employed :

Tum ipsum recondendum est ; ac, si id manus facere non potest, vulsella quali fabri utuntur iniicienda est, recte se habenti capiti ab ea parte qua sima est ; ut ea parte qua gibba est eminens os in suam sedem compellat.

' Then it is to be replaced, and if that cannot be done by hand the forceps such as smiths use is to be inserted, the head being kept straight by the snub-nosed part so that the curved part forces the bone into position.'

The blacksmith's tongs is very frequently represented in ancient art. Pl. XLII, fig. 2 shows a forceps from Roman London in the Guildhall Museum.

Tooth and Stump Forceps.

Greek, ὀδοντάγρα, ῥιζάγρα.

The ancients regarded tooth extraction as an operation to

be avoided wherever possible. Caelius Aurelianus says death had followed in some cases, and that in the temple of Apollo at Delos there hung a tooth forceps of lead as a reminder for operators to exert little force in tooth extraction (*Pass. Tard.* II. iv). Scribonius Largus (*Comp.* liii) is equally pessimistic :

Ad dentium dolorem quamvis plurimi dicant forcipes remedium esse, multa tamen citra hanc necessitatem scio profuisse.

Celsus (VII. xii) says extraction may result in injury to the temples and eyes, and fracture or dislocation of the jaw may occur. He recommends therefore to free the tooth all round down to the socket, then to shake it repeatedly till it has been thoroughly loosened, and remove it with fingers or forceps. If the tooth be hollow, it should be plugged with lint or lead to prevent it breaking under the forceps. The tooth should be pulled out straight, lest the alveolus be broken. Stumps are to be removed with the forceps which the Greeks call ῥιζάγρα. Paulus Aegineta (VI. xxvii) bids us scarify down to the socket and loosen the tooth gradually by shaking with a tooth extractor (ὀδοντάγρα) and extract it. Supernumerary teeth are, if fast, to be rasped down with a graving tool ; if loose, to be extracted with tooth forceps (διὰ τῆς ὀδοντάγρας). There is no ancient forceps which can with certainty be set down as a tooth forceps, although some have looked upon the Pompeian forceps (see p. 135) as a tooth extractor. Although its shape is not otherwise unsuitable for this purpose its jaws are not particularly well adapted for seizing a tooth, as they are not hollowed inside. It may be noted that the tooth forceps was evidently a 'universal', as no special variety is ever mentioned beyond the two I have given—'tooth' and 'stump'. Whatever the shape of the Graeco-Roman forceps was it seems to have been a handy instrument for many different manipulations. Soranus (ii. 63) says that in impaction of the foetal cranium we may open the head and remove the bones with a bone forceps or a tooth forceps (ὀστάγρας ἢ ὀδοντάγρας). Paul (VI. xc) says that in fracture of the skull the fragment is to be surrounded with perforations by the drill and finally separated with chisels, the chips being removed with the fingers or with tooth forceps, bone forceps, &c. (ὀδοντάγρα ἢ ὀστάγρα). Again in ch. lxxxviii he says that if the shaft of a weapon imbedded in the flesh be broken off, the weapon may be extracted with a tooth forceps or a stump forceps (ὀδοντάγρας ἢ ῥιζάγρας).

Tooth Elevator.

In a note on a passage in Hippocrates describing the lever for replacing the protruding end of a fractured bone, Galen mentions an instrument for levering teeth. He says the instruments for levering the bone are of the same size as the instrument for levering teeth (xviii. 593). As we know from Paul (VI. cvi) that these bone levers were seven or eight finger breadths in length, we may take this as the length of the tooth elevator.

Tooth Scalers.

Greek, ξυστήριον, σμιλίον, σμιλιωτόν (sc. ὄργανον); Latin, *scalper medicinalis*.

Paul (VI. xxviii) mentions a small raspatory used for removing tartar from teeth :

'The scaly concretions which adhere to teeth we may remove with the scoop of a specillum, or with a scaler (ξυστηρίῳ) or a file.'

Scribonius Largus (*Comp.* liii) mentions an excavator :

Itaque cum etiam exesus est aliqua ex parte, tum non suadeo protinus tollendum, sed excidendum scalpro medicinali, qua cavatus est, quod sine ullo fit dolore, reliqua enim solida pars eius et speciem et usum dentis praestabit.

Marcellus conveys this passage entire (*De Med.* xii).

Paul (VI. xii) says supernumerary teeth may be cut down with excavators (τῶν σμιλιωτῶν).

File.

Greek, ῥινάριον, ῥίνη, ῥινίον; Latin, *lima, limula.*

In compound fracture with protrusion of bone Celsus says :

'Should any small piece of bone protrude, if it is blunt it should be reduced to its place. If it is sharp its point should first be cut off if it is long, and if short it should be filed. "In either case it should be smoothed with the raspatory."' (Si longius est, praecidendum; si brevius, limandum, et utrumque scalpro laevandum.)

The application of the raspatory to smooth the bone after the use of the file shows that it must have been more of the nature of a rasp than a file which was used for bones. Scribonius Largus speaks of a wood file or rasp used in reducing a hart's horn to powder (*Comp.* cxli):

Ad lumbricos satis commode facit et santonica herba, quae non viget, et cornum cervinum limatum lima lignaria.

Files were largely used in dental work. All the surgeons state that where a tooth projects above its fellows it should be filed down; Galen says that for this purpose he has invented an olivary pointed file of steel: σιδήριον ἐποίησα ῥινίον πυρηνοειδές (xiv. 871).

Aetius copies Galen's chapter word for word (II. iv. 30). Paul (VI. xxviii) says the file (ῥινάριον) may be used to remove tartar from teeth.

There are several files of steel in the Naples Museum which are classed among the surgical instruments. Many Roman files of steel which have been found in London are now in the Guildhall Museum. Some of these have transverse edges like our own files. Other extant specimens have coarse frets on them, like our wood rasps. Pl. XLII, fig. 1 shows one in the Guildhall collection, which is of the rasp variety.

Forceps for extracting Weapons.

Greek, βελουλκόν (sc. ὄργανον).

Paul has a most interesting chapter on the extraction of

weapons, and in it he mentions a special instrument for extracting weapons, evidently a forceps :

' If the head of the weapon has fixed in the flesh, it is to be drawn out with the hands, or by laying hold of the appendage which is called the shaft, if it has not fallen off. This part is commonly made of wood. When it has fallen off we make the extraction by means of a tooth forceps, or a stump forceps, or a forceps for extracting weapons (βελουλκοῦ), or any other convenient instrument. And sometimes we make an incision in the flesh around it in the first place, if the wound do not admit the instrument ' (VI. lxxxvii).

It is true that etymologically we are only entitled to translate βελουλκοῦ by ' weapon-extractor ', but its association with the other two forceps shows pretty conclusively that a forceps is meant, and Celsus says weapons are to be extracted with the forceps under similar conditions. In the picture of Aeneas wounded, found in a house at Stabiae and now in the Naples Museum, the surgeon, Iapix, is engaged in extracting a weapon from the wound in the thigh of the hero. The instrument he is using is a long forceps with crossed legs (Pl. XLIV).

Periosteal Elevator for the Pericranium.

Greek, ὑποσπαθιστήρ, σπαθιστήρ.

The hypospathister was an elevator for separating the pericranium from the calvarium. It gave the name to a formidable operation in which it was used, viz. hypospathismus. This operation is described by Galen, Aetius, and Paul, by the latter (VI. vi) best of all. Paul is the only one who mentions the instrument by name. The operation consisted in making three vertical incisions, one down each side of the forehead and one down the centre. Next the skin was raised along with the pericranium from the whole of the front of the forehead with the hypospathister (ὑποσπαθιστήρ), and the vessels lying in the raised flaps were subcutaneously divided by a knife passed under them, with its back to the skull. The elevator by which the pericranium was separated is called by Paul ὑποσπαθιστήρ. The operation is mentioned by Epiphanius, a bishop of Alexandria in the fourth century, by whom the instrument is referred to as σπαθιστήρ.

Impellent.

Greek, διωστήρ.

In his chapter on the extraction of weapons, one of the most remarkable chapters in the whole of his works, Paul mentions an impellent for forcing an arrow head through a part so as to extract it at the side opposite to that by which it went in.

'If the head of the weapon has passed to the other side and it is found impossible to extract it by the way it entered, having divided the parts opposite we extract it through the middle of them, either extracting it in the manner spoken of (i. e. with forceps), or we make an opening by means of the weapon itself, pushing it by the shaft, or, if that has come away, by an impellent instrument (διωστῆρος), taking care not to divide a nerve, artery, vein, or any important part; for it would be malpractice if, in extracting the weapon, we should do more mischief than the weapon itself had done. If the weapon has a tang, which is ascertained by examination with the probe, having introduced the female part of the impellent instrument and engaged it, we push the weapon forwards, or, if it has a socket, the male part' (τὴν θήλειαν τοῦ διωστῆρος καθέντες καὶ ἐναρμόσαντες ὠθήσομεν τὸ βέλος εἰ δὲ αὐλὸν τὸν ἄρρενα).

Impellents formed an important part of the armamentarium of the surgeon, at least down to the time of Scultetus, and in his works and in those of Albucasis and Paré there are numerous figures of these instruments. None of these quite agree with the idea of the instrument which one gathers from Paul's description. It would seem to have been a very simple affair, probably a plain rod of metal pointed at one end and hollowed at the other, the pointed end being introduced into the socket of an arrow where it possessed one, the hollow end being fitted over the tip of the tang in cases where the arrow was tanged.

Arrow Scoop.

Greek, κυαθίσκος Διοκλεῖος.

A scoop for extracting arrow heads is thus described by Celsus (VII. v):

Latum vero telum, si conditum est, ab altera parte educi non expedit, ne ingenti vulneri ipsi quoque ingens vulnus adiiciamus. Evellendum est ergo genere quodam ferramenti quod Διοκλείου κυαθίσκον Graeci vocant, quoniam auctorem Dioclem habet: quem inter priscos maximosque medicos fuisse iam posui. Lamina, vel ferrea vel etiam aenea, ab altero capite duos utrimque deorsum conversos uncos habet; ab altero duplicata lateribus, leviterque extrema in eam partem inclinata quae sinuata est, insuper ibi etiam perforata est. Haec iuxta telum transversa demittitur; deinde ubi ad imum mucronem ventum est paulum torquetur, ut telum foramine suo excipiat; quum in cavo mucro est, duo digiti subiecti partis alterius uncis simul et ferramentum id extrahunt et telum.

' But a broad weapon if buried should not be extracted from a counter opening, lest to one large wound we add another; therefore it is to be extracted with a special variety of instrument which the Greeks call the Scoop of Diocles, since Diocles invented it. I have already stated that he was one of the most eminent of the old practitioners. Its blade of iron, or even of bronze, has at one end two hooks, one at each side turned backwards. At the other end it is folded over at the sides, and the end is slightly curved up towards that part which is bent. Moreover in it there is a perforation. This is introduced crosswise near the weapon, then when it comes near the point it is twisted a little so that it receives the point in the hole. When the weapon is in the cavity two fingers placed under the hooks at the other end simultaneously extract both the instrument and the weapon.'

This description seems very definite until we attempt to reconstruct the instrument, when it becomes evident that more than one construction may be put on some parts of it. Pl. XLV, fig. 4, shows the instrument as conceived by me.

CHAPTER IX

BLADDER AND GYNAECOLOGICAL INSTRUMENTS

Catheter.

THE catheter is very frequently referred to. Galen (xiv. 787) thus describes it:

'When urine is not passed on account of excessive dilatation of the bladder so that it cannot contract, we draw off the urine with a catheter. Therefore an instrument like the Roman letter S is let down into the bladder by the urethra. A thread is passed into it which has in its tip a little wool dipped in urine. Then it is drawn out and the urine follows it like a guide.'

This method of preparing the catheter and the reasons for so doing are discussed at somewhat greater length in the following selection from Paul (VI. xix):

'Wherefore taking a catheter proportionate to the age and sex we prepare the instrument for use. The mode of preparation is this: having bound a little wool round with a thread and introduced the thread by means of a sharp rush into the pipe of the catheter, and having cut off the projecting parts of the wool with a pair of scissors, we put the catheter into oil. Having then placed the patient on a convenient seat and used fomentation, if there be no contra-indication we take the catheter and introduce it direct down to the base of the penis, then we must draw the penis up to the umbilicus (for at this part there is a bend in the passage), and in this position push the instrument onwards. When in the perinaeum it approaches the anus we must bend the penis with the instrument in it down to its natural position, for from the perinaeum to the bladder the passage is upwards, and we must push the instrument onwards till we reach the cavity of the bladder. We afterwards take out the thread fastened into the opening of the catheter, in order that the urine, being attracted by the wool, may follow as happens in syphons.'

It is occasionally, in cases of cancer of the prostate, of service to adopt this proceeding to prevent the eye of the catheter from getting blocked before the bladder is entered, but it is strange that Galen should have fallen into the mistake of thinking that it is necessary to set up a syphon action, as he was well aware of the expulsive power possessed by the bladder; in fact, his explanation of the physiology of urination is almost up to date.

Celsus gives a good description of the catheter both male and female (VII. xxvi):

Res vero interdum cogit emoliri manu urinam, quum illa non redditur, aut quia senectute iter eius collapsum est, aut quia calculus vel concretum aliquid ex sanguine intus se opposuit: ac mediocris quoque inflammatio saepe eam reddi naturaliter prohibet. Idque non in viris tantummodo, sed in feminis quoque interdum necessarium est. Ergo aeneae fistulae fiunt; quae ut omni corpori ampliori minorique sufficiant, ad mares tres, ad feminas duae medico habendae sunt; ex virilibus maxima decem et quinque digitorum, media duodecim, minima novem, ex muliebribus maior novem, minor sex. Incurvas vero esse eas paulum, sed magis viriles, oportet, laevesque admodum; ac neque nimis plenas neque nimis tenues.

There are fine specimens of the catheter, both male and female, in the Naples Museum. The male catheter is from the ' House of the Physician' in Pompeii. It is 24 cm. in length and is about the size of a No. 11 English. It has two gentle curves, so that it closely resembles the instrument reintroduced by Petit in the eighteenth century. See Pl. XLV, fig. 1. A catheter of similar shape, but broken in three pieces, was found by some workmen at Baden in the Seventies. They were given by Dr. Wagner, of Baden, to Mr. Atkinson, M.P., London, and are possibly now in some English collection (Brunner, *op. cit.* p. 42).

In the excavation of the Roman Military Hospital at Baden, 1893, a fragment of a catheter was found, and is now in the possession of M. Kellersberger. It consists of the curved part of a catheter, and it is 13 cm. long and about the size of a No. 10 English. The curve is considerably greater than that of the Naples specimen (Un Hôpital Militaire Romain, planche ix).

The female catheter in the Naples Museum is 0·98 m. long, and of the same diameter as the male one. It is straight (Pl. XLV, fig. 2)

Bladder Sounds.

Had the ancients solid bladder sounds? They must have been well aware of the characteristic grating sensation conveyed to the skilled hand on striking a stone with a metal instrument, for we have several references in the classics to the manœuvre of pushing back, by means of a catheter, a stone impacted in the urethra. Rufus of Ephesus (Περὶ λιθιώσης κύστεως) says of impacted urethral calculus : 'Those that are stuck fast push back with the catheter if you prefer not to do lithotomy' (ἐρείδοντας οὖν εἰ μὴ θέλοις τέμνειν ἀπῶσαι τῷ αὐλίσκῳ). Soranus (II. xviii) says if a stone is the cause of dystocia we must push it out of the neck of the bladder into the bladder with a catheter (καθετήρ). The word Rufus uses puts it beyond doubt that a hollow tube is meant, or we might have argued that καθετήρ did not necessarily mean a hollow tube, since Hippocrates uses it in the sense of a uterine plug (ii. 830). Yet strange to say, the sensation conveyed to the hand and ear on striking a stone with a metal instrument is nowhere definitely given as a cardinal symptom by a classical writer.

Rufus describes the symptoms of vesical calculus at length and finishes with instructions for searching the bladder. The word he uses (μήλωσις) at first sight seems to indicate that this was done with a sound, but it turns out to be bimanual rectal examination only which he describes. The use of the sound as a staff in lithotomy, or as a dilator of a strictured urethra, was not known to the ancients, and thus we have no evidence from the literature that a solid bougie existed. Some instruments have come down to us, however, which seem undoubted solid bladder sounds.

There are three sounds of bronze in the Naples Museum, which have the identical appearance of our modern bladder sounds. It might be argued that these have not quite the shape of the catheter described by the ancients, but there is an instrument in the Mainz Museum against which even this objection cannot be brought. It is a solid sound of the double curvature described by Celsus, and is identical in shape with the catheter from the Pompeian surgeon's house (Pl. XLV, fig. 3).

Lithotomy Scoop.

Greek, λιθουλκός ; Latin, *uncus, ferramentum quo in sectione calculus protrahitur.*

Celsus thus describes the extraction of calculus through a perineal incision by means of a lithotomy scoop :

Quum vero ea patefacta est, in conspectum calculus venit ; in cuius colore nullum discrimen est. Ipse si exiguus est, digitis ab altera parte propelli, ab altera protrahi potest ; si maior, iniiciendus a superiore parte uncus est, eius rei causa factus. Is est ad extremum tenuis, in semicirculi speciem retusae latitudinis ; ab exteriore parte laevis, qua corpori iungitur ; ab interiore asper, qua calculum attingit. Isque longior potius esse debet ; nam brevis extrahendi vim non habet. Ubi iniectus est in utrumque latus inclinandus est, ut appareat an calculus teneatur ; quia si apprehensus est, ille simul inclinatur.

'When it is opened there comes into view the calculus, the colour of which is unmistakeable. If it is small it is to be pushed by the fingers from one side and pulled from the other. If too large the hook for the purpose is to be put in above it. The hook is slender at the end and flattened out in the shape of a semicircle, smooth externally where it comes in contact with the tissues, rough internally where it meets the calculus. The hook should be pretty long, for a short one has no power of extraction. When it has been inserted it should be inclined to either side, so that it may be seen whether the calculus is caught, because if it is held it also is inclined to the side' (VII. xxvii).

The above passage gives a very complete account of the lithotomy scoop. The only thing it leaves undecided is the

breadth.   Was it a broad, spoon-like scoop, or was it a hook-
like instrument ?   That the latter was the case is proved by
the following passage also from Celsus (VII. xxvi):

Nonnunquam etiam prolapsus in ipsam fistulam calculus :
quia subinde ea extenuatur non longe ab exitu inhaerescit.
Eum, si fieri potest, oportet evellere vel oriculario specillo,
vel eo ferramento quo in sectione calculus protrahitur.

'Sometimes also a stone slips into the urethra itself and
lodges near the meatus, because at that part there is a con-
striction.   It should if possible be extracted either with an
ear probe, or with the instrument for the extraction of
calculus in lithotomy.'

This shows that the scoop must have been quite a narrow
instrument, or it could not have passed into the urethra.
It must have had very much the same appearance as the
modern 'Ferguson's Scoop '.   We have two extant specimens
of the ancient lithotomy scoop in the Naples Museum, one
of which is shown in Pl. IV; and in the marble *ex voto*
tablet in the Athens Museum, to which I have already
referred, there is a representation of a manubriolus curved
so as to serve as a lithotomy scoop (Pl. XLVI, fig. 2).
Rufus of Ephesus mentions this form of scalpel handle.

Lithotomy Forceps.

Was there a forceps for extracting calculus from the
bladder?   The sixteenth-century translation of Aetius (IV.
iv. 94) by Cornarius has the following passage, under the
treatment of calculus in the female :

Et tunc paululum supra pudendi alas, quo loco calculus
occurrit sectionem facito et per calcularium forcipem ex-
trahito.

The original Greek of this part of Aetius has not yet been
published, but from a pretty intimate knowledge of Cornarius's methods I have a strong suspicion that 'calcularium
forcipem ' may be a free translation of λιθουλκός, as in the
following passage in Paul :

'Sometimes from the pressure of the finger or fingers at
the anus the stone starts out readily at the same time as

the incision is made, without requiring extraction. But if it does not of itself start out we must extract it with the instrument called the stone extractor' (τοῦ λιθουλκοῦ) (VI. lx).

Adams translates λιθουλκός by 'forceps for extracting stone ', but this is not quite a justifiable translation. The instruments whose names end in -ουλκός, and which are derived from ἕλκω, are certainly in many instances forceps, e. g. βελουλκός, a forceps for extracting weapons, but in other cases they are as certainly not. I need only refer to ἐμβρυουλκός, which is conclusively described as a hook for extracting the dead foetus. Thus while it is possible that the λιθουλκός may have been a forceps, the etymology of the word does not entitle us to translate by any term more definite than 'stone extractor'. Galen (xiv. 787) uses the word λιθολάβος, which has a more definite meaning. The majority of words compounded of -λάβος means some variety of forceps, e. g. σαρκολάβος, tumour vulsellum. The etymological evidence thus leaves the matter open, with a slight balance in favour of there having been a forceps. I should have had no hesitation in translating λιθολάβος to mean a forceps, had it not been that Celsus evidently had no cognizance of a stone forceps. Galen, however, lived after Celsus, and we may note that the Arabians used such an instrument. Albucasis says that if the stone does not start out it must be seized with a forceps or a hook, and failing removal by these means it is to be broken up with forceps. One forceps in the Naples Museum, from the house of the physician, seems to be suited for the operation (Pl. XLVI, fig. 3). The handles are short in proportion to the blades, and it seems better suited to grasp some substance inside the bow than between the jaws. The unfinished condition of the tips of the handles indicates that they had been inserted into handles of wood.

Lithotrite.

Latin, *ferramentum.*

A sort of chisel by which a calculus was split is thus described by Celsus:

Si quando autem is maior non videtur nisi rupta cervice extrahi posse, findendus est; cuius repertor Ammonius ob id λιθοτόμος cognominatus est.   Id hoc modo fit: uncus iniicitur calculo sic ut facile eum concussum quoque teneat, ne is retro revolvatur; tum ferramentum adhibetur crassitudinis modicae, prima parte tenui, sed retusa, quod admotum calculo, et ex altera parte ictum, eum findit.

' If at any time it seems too large and impossible to be extracted without splitting the cervix, it is to be split. The originator of this is Ammonius, hence called the lithotomist. It is performed in this manner. A scoop is put over the calculus in such a way that it easily holds it even when struck from sliding back; then there is applied an instrument of moderate thickness, slender at the tip, but blunt, which being placed against the calculus and struck on the other end splits it ' (VII. xxvi).

The above paragraph really gives us all the information we possess about the instrument.   It is evidently a slender chisel.   A passage in Aretaeus (*Morb. Chron.* ii. 9) is held by some to refer to lithotripsy (digital). The reading, however, is dubious.

Rectal Speculum.

Greek, ἑδροδιαστολεύς, μικρὸν διόπτριον, κατοπτήρ.

The earliest mention of the rectal speculum is to be found in the treatise on fistula by Hippocrates:

῞Υπτιον κατακλίνας τὸν ἄνθρωπον κατοπτῆρι κατιδὼν τὸ διαβε-βρωμένον τοῦ ἀρχοῦ.

' Laying the patient on his back and examining the ulcerated part of the bowel by means of the rectal speculum ' (iii. 331).

Again, a little further on, he mentions its use in the treatment of piles ; and Paul (VI. lxxviii) says:

' With regard to blind fistulae Leonidas says: " We dilate the anus, as we do the female vagina, with the anal or small speculum " ' (τῷ ἑδροδιαστολεῖ (τῷ μικρῷ διοπτρίῳ λέγω) διαστεῖλαι τὴν ἕδραν ὡς γυναικεῖον κόλπον).

There is a rectal speculum in the Naples Museum (No. 78,031). It is a two-bladed instrument, working with a hinge

in the middle. It is 0·15 m. in length, and the greatest
stretch of the blades is 0·07 m. It represents an instrument
used to dilate the vagina as well as the rectum, and got its
name ' small dilator ' in contradistinction to the other vaginal
speculum, which we shall see was worked by a screw, and
was called the speculum magnum. The rectal speculum
was also called κατοπτήρ, in contradistinction to the vaginal
speculum which was called διόπτρα. In Galen's Lexicon
they are explained as follows:

Κατοπτῆρι, τῷ καλουμένῳ ἑδροδιαστολεῖ, ὥσπερ γε καὶ διόπτρα ὁ
γυναικῶν διαστολεύς.

' The catopter, which is called the anal dilator, in the same
way as the diopter is called the female dilator.'

Pl. XLVI, fig. 1 shows one of two similar rectal specula
from Pompeii (Naples Museum).

Vaginal Speculum.

Greek, διόπτρα ; Latin, *speculum magnum matricis* (late).

Soranus is the first author who makes mention of the
speculum specially made for the vagina. The original
Greek of this chapter of Soranus is lost, but we have a
Latin translation of it preserved to us by Moschion. The
heading of this chapter in Soranus, which was No. xxxiv,
was Περὶ διοπτρισμοῦ. I shall give part of this chapter from
Moschion :

Qua Disciplina Organo aperiendae sint Mulieres.

Scio me retro ad inspiciendam altitudinem mulieris frequentius organi mentionem fecisse quod Graecitas dioptran
vocat. Et quoniam nisi insinuata fuerit disciplina quatenus
hoc ipsud fieri possit, occurrente necessitate obstetrices facere
non audent, idcirco placuit nobis ut etiam hoc gynaeciis
adderemus, ut ex rebus huic corpori necessariis nihil dimi-
sisse videamur. Itaque supinam iactans eam quae inspici
habet, accipies fasciam longam et in media parte eius
duobus laqueis factis, ita ut inter se cubitum unum habeant
laquei illi, duabus vero manibus mulieris missis, medietatem
quae interest cervici eius inducis. Deinde reliqua fasciae
sub anquilas missa ad manus alligabis, ita ut patefacti pedes
ventri eius cohaereant. Deinde accepto organo et uncto
priapisco, quem Graeci loton dicunt, in aliquantum ad prunas

calefacere (debes), deinde sine quassatione priapiscum inicere, susum scilicet axe posito, iubere etiam ministro ut
aperiendo organo axem torquere incipiat, ut paulatim
partes ipsae aperiantur. Cum vero post visum organo
tollere volueris, ministro iubere ut iterum axem torqueat
quo organum claudi possit, ita tamen ut cum adhuc in
aliquantum patet sic auferatur, ne universa clusura aliquas
teneat et nocere incipiat.

We have also preserved by Paul a chapter by Archigenes
on abscess of the womb (VI. lxxiii), in which the different
parts of the speculum are again named, and from it also we
learn that there were different sizes of the instrument proportioned to suit different ages. The patient having been
fixed in the lithotomy position in the manner described by
Soranus :

'The operator is to make the examination with a speculum
(διόπτρα) proportioned to the age of the patient. The person
using the speculum should measure with a probe the depth
of the woman's vagina, lest the priapiscus of the speculum
(τοῦ τῆς διόπτρας λωτοῦ) being too long it should happen that the
uterus be pressed on. If it be ascertained that the tube is
longer than the woman's vagina, folded compresses are to be
laid on the labia in order that the speculum may be laid on
them. The priapiscus is to be introduced while the screw
(τὸν κοχλίον) is uppermost. The speculum is to be held by
the operator. The screw is to be turned by the assistant,
so that the blades of the tube (τῶν ἐμπλησμάτων τοῦ λωτοῦ)
being separated, the vagina may be expanded.'

We have little difficulty in recognizing among the instruments found in Pompeii three of the vaginal specula referred to in these passages. All are excellent specimens
of the instrument maker's skill. They are in the Naples
Museum. The first discovered (No. 78,030) was found in
the house of the physician at Pompeii. The blades are at
right angles to the instrument (Pl. XLVII), and when
closed form a tube the size of the thumb. On turning the
screw a cross-bar forces the two upper blades outwards, till
sufficient dilation is got for operative purposes. The
diameter of the tube at its maximum of expansion is

0·09 m. The whole instrument is 0·23 m. long. Another instrument on a similar principle but with a quadrivalve priapiscus was discovered in 1882 (Pl. XLIX). It is 0·315 m. long. It is now fixed by oxidation, so that the blades cannot be moved. On turning the screw the lower blades could be drawn downwards, at the same time separating slightly, while the upper blades diverged also (No. 113,264 Naples Mus.). Lately a third, similar to that shown in Pl. XLVII, has been found in Pompeii. Note that the screw in the three-bladed instrument is a left-handed one. That in the four-bladed instrument is right-handed. This causes right-handed motion to open the instrument in either case. There is, however, an instrument similar to these trivalve instruments in the museum at Athens. It differs in having the screw right-handed (Pl. XLVIII). Mr. Bosanquet, late of the British Institute of Archaeology at Athens, was kind enough to procure me a photograph of this instrument, but he tells me that there is no satisfactory account of its provenance and its authenticity is doubtful. It seems possible that it is a copy of one of the Naples specimens by some one who has omitted to observe that the screw in these is left-handed.

Traction Hook for Embryo.

Greek, ἐμβρυουλκός ; Latin, *uncus.*

Celsus has an interesting chapter on the removal of the foetus in difficult labour. He says (VII. xxix):

Tum, si caput proximum est, demitti debet uncus undique laevis, acuminis brevis, qui vel oculo, vel auri, vel ori, interdum etiam fronti recte iniicitur; deinde attractus infantem educit. Neque tamen quolibet is tempore extrahi debet. Nam, si compresso vulvae ore id tentatum est, non emittente eo, infans abrumpitur, et unci acumen in ipsum os vulvae delabitur; sequiturque nervorum distentio, et ingens periculum mortis. Igitur, compressa vulva, conquiescere; hiante, leniter trahere oportet; et per has occasiones paulatim eum educere. Trahere autem dextra manus uncum; sinistra intus posita infantem ipsum, simulque dirigere eum debet.

'Then if the head presents there ought to be inserted a hook, smooth all round, with a short point which is properly fixed in the eye or the ear or the mouth, sometimes even in the forehead, which being drawn on extracts the child. Nor is it to be drawn on without regard to circumstance. For if the attempt is made with an undilated cervix, not getting exit the foetus is broken up, and the point of the hook catches on the cervix and inflammation follows and much danger of death. Therefore, it is necessary with a contracted cervix to wait quietly, with a dilated one to make gentle traction, and during these times to extract it gradually. The right hand ought to make the traction on the hook, the left place inside to draw the child and at the same time to direct it.'

The following passage in Soranus shows that it was customary also to insert a second hook opposite the first and to make traction on both at the same time:

'The best places for the insertion of the hooks are in head presentations, the eyes, the occiput, and the mouth, the clavicles, and the parts about the ribs. In footling cases the pubes, ribs, and clavicles, are the best. Warm oil having been applied as a lubricant the hook is to be held in the right hand ; the curvature concealed in the left hand is to be carefully introduced into the uterus, and plunged into some of the places mentioned till it pierce right through to the hollow part beneath. Then a second one is to be put in opposite to it (καταπείρειν δὲ καὶ ἀντίθετον τούτῳ δεύτερον), in order that the pulling may be straight and not one-sided' (II. xix).

Aetius (IV. iv. 23) and Paul (VI. lxxiv) copy this.

Hippocrates (ii. 701) bids us break up the head with a cephalotribe in such a way as not to splinter the bones, and remove the bones with bone forceps; or, a traction hook (τῷ ἑλκυστῆρι) being inserted near the clavicle so as to hold, make traction but not much at once, but little by little, withdrawing and again inserting it.

There are three traction hooks from Pompeii in the Naples Museum. One of these is given in Pl. L, fig. 1. They are of steel, with handles of bronze. Hooks on the same principle, and differing in appearance very little from the Pompeian hooks, are still used by veterinary surgeons.

Decapitator.

Of transverse presentations, Celsus says :

Remedio est cervix praecisa; ut separatim utraque pars auferatur. Id unco fit, qui, priori similis, in interiore tantum parte per totam aciem exacuitur. Tum id agendum est ut ante caput deinde reliqua pars auferatur.

'The treatment is to divide the neck so that each part may be extracted separately. This is done with a hook which, though similar to the last, is sharpened on its inside only, along its whole border. Then we must endeavour to bring away the head first, and then the rest of the body.'

Decapitation has now given way before Caesarean section ; but the decapitator, little altered since the days of Celsus, still finds a place in surgical instrument catalogues.

Paul and Aetius both mention division at the neck, but do not describe a special instrument. A ring knife for dismembering the foetus has already been discussed among the cutting instruments ; but this seems to be a different variety with a handle, which it is convenient to discuss in proximity to the embryo hook. Pl. L, fig. 2 shows a knife on this principle in the Bibliothèque Nationale.

Cranioclast.

Greek, πίεστρον, ἐμβρυοθλάστης, θλάστης ;

The cranioclast is mentioned by Hippocrates (ii. 701).

Σχίσαντα τὴν κεφαλὴν μαχαιρίῳ ξυμπλάσαι ἵνα μὴ θραύσῃ τῷ πιέστρῳ καὶ τὰ ὀστέα ἕλκειν τῷ ὀστεουλκῷ.

'Opening the head with a scalpel, break it up with the cranioclast in such a way as not to splinter it into fragments, and remove the bones with a bone forceps.'

The nature of the cranioclast is pretty well indicated by this passage, and in Galen's Lexicon we find πιέστρῳ defined as τῷ ἐμβρυοθλάστῃ καλουμένῳ. I give drawings from Albucasis of a 'forceps to crush the child's head' (Pl. LI, fig. 3).

Cephalotribe.

Whether or not the instrument last described was used also for the operation of cephalotripsy, or whether there was a special instrument, we cannot say, but it is certain that the operation of crushing the head and delivering the child without removing the bones was practised.   In Aetius (IV. iv. 23) cephalotripsy is thus described:

'But if the foetus be doubled on itself and cannot be straightened, if the head is presenting, break up the bones of it without cutting the skin.   Then to some part of it fix on a traction hook and make traction, and the legs becoming straightened out we get it away.'

Though there is an essential difference between the operations of cephalotripsy and cranioclasie there is no essential difference between the instruments necessary for carrying out the same, and it is possible that the instrument used may be the same as the last.   The cephalotribe figured by Albucasis is not essentially different from his cranioclast (see Pl. LI, fig. 4).

Midwifery Forceps.

Had the Greeks and Romans a forceps for extracting the child alive?   Probably not.   We have no mention of any such instrument by Soranus or Paul, both accomplished obstetricians, nor can any description of such an instrument be found in the voluminous pseudo-Hippocratic works on women.   Adams, in a note to Paul, III. lxxvi, says that though the Roman and Greek writers do not mention the forceps, Avicenna does so, and he says that a forceps was dug up in the house of an obstetrix at Pompeii bearing a considerable resemblance to the modern forceps.   The only passage I have met with in the slightest degree supporting the notion that the ancients ever delivered the child alive with instruments is one in the pseudo-Hippocratic treatise *De Superfoetatione*, where we are told that:

'If the woman has a difficult labour, and the child delay long in the passage and be born not easily but with difficulty and with the mechanical aids (μηχαναῖς) of the physician, such children are of weak vitality, and the umbilical cord should not be cut till they make water or sneeze or cry' (i. 465).

We are not entitled to translate μηχαναῖς by 'instruments', because it may mean any mechanical aid such as a fillet, or even assistance with the fingers of the accoucheur; but, even granting that it refers to instruments, it might mean no more than, e. g., the embryo hooks already described. With them, terrible as they were, the child must frequently have been born alive, though mutilated. A child would have had a far better chance of being born alive with them than with the murderously toothed forceps of Albucasis (Pl. XLI, figs. 3, 4), with which probably no child could have been born alive. As regards the statement that Avicenna knew of the forceps, his directions are that the fillet is to be applied, and, if that fail, the forceps is to be put on and the child extracted with it. If that fail, the child is to be extracted by incision, as in the case of a dead foetus. This passage, says Adams, puts it beyond doubt that the Arabians were acquainted with the method of extracting the child alive with the forceps.

This is, however, not quite correct. A full consideration of Avicenna's words seems to me to lead to the conclusion that he is describing no more than extraction with a craniotomy forceps. If the forceps fail the child is to be extracted by incision, as in the case of a foetus already dead (and decomposed so that the forceps would not hold).

As regards Adams' statement that a forceps like ours was dug up in Pompeii one may ask, 'Where is that forceps now?' It is certainly not in the Naples Museum, where all the finds from Herculaneum and Pompeii have been stored since the excavations were commenced. Adams has probably been misled by some notice of the 'Pompeian forceps' (Pl. XLIII), which many consider adapted for removing the cranial bones when the child's head is broken up in cephalotripsy. It is, however, a sequestrum forceps.

Uterine Curette.

Hippocrates (ed. Van der Linden, vol. ii, p. 394) says :

If the menses form thrombi . . . we must wind the skin of a vulture or a piece of vellum round a curette and curette the os uteri (καὶ περὶ ξύστραν περιειλίξας γυπὸς δέρμα ἢ ὑμένα, διαξύειν τὸ στόμα τῶν μητρέων).

ξύστρα may of course mean the strigil, and some forms of strigil, such as the one shown in Pl. XXV, fig. 1, are not ill adapted for the purpose.

Instrument for destroying foetus in utero.

Greek, ἐμβρυοσφάκτης ; Latin, aeneum spiculum.

Apart from the destruction of the foetus in criminal abortion, which was so common at Rome in the time of the Empire, we have mention of an instrument for legitimately producing the death of the foetus from humane motives before forced delivery. It is mentioned by Tertullian in his sermon De Anima, and the passage is so interesting that I give it in full. It is, moreover, an example of the unexpected places in which information regarding the surgery of the ancients crops up. Tertullian is arguing that the foetus is alive in utero, and does not, as others hold, simply take on life in the act of birth, and to support his conclusions he uses the following argument :

Denique et mortui eduntur quomodo, nisi et vivi? qui autem et mortui, nisi qui prius vivi? Atquin et in ipso adhuc utero infans trucidatur necessaria crudelitate, quum in exitu obliquatus denegat partum ; matricida, ni moriturus. Itaque et inter arma medicorum et organon est, quo prius patescere secreta coguntur tortili temperamento, cum anulo cultrato, quo intus membra caeduntur anxio arbitrio, cum hebete unco, quo totum facinus extrahitur violento puerperio. Est etiam aeneum spiculum, quo iugulatio ipsa dirigitur caeco latrocinio ; ἐμβρυοσφάκτην appellant de infanticidii officio, utique viventis infantis peremptorium. Hoc et Hippocrates habuit et Asclepiades et Erasistratus et

maiorum quoque prosector Herophilus et mitior ipse
Soranus, certi animal esse conceptum, atque ita miserti
infelicissimae huiusmodi infantiae, ut prius occidatur ne
viva lanietur.

' Finally there are cases of children that are dead when
they are born, how so unless they have also lived? For
who are dead unless they have previously been alive? And
yet, an infant is sometimes by an act of necessary cruelty
destroyed when yet in the womb, when owing to an oblique
presentation at birth delivery is made impossible and the
child would cause the death of the mother unless it were
doomed itself to die. And accordingly there is among the
appliances of medical men an instrument by which the
private parts are dilated with a priapiscus worked by
a screw, and also a ring-knife whereby the limbs are cut
off in the womb with judicious care, and a blunt hook by
which the whole mass is extracted and a violent form of
delivery in this way effected. There is also a bronze stylet
with which a secret death is inflicted; they call it the
ἐμβρυοσφάκτης (foeticide) from its use in infanticide, as being
fatal to a living infant. Hippocrates had this (instrument),
Asclepiades and Erasistratus, and of the ancients also
Herophilus the anatomist, and Soranus, a man of gentler
character. Who, being assured that a living thing had been
conceived, mercifully judged that an unfortunate infant of
this sort should be destroyed before birth to save it from
being mangled alive.'

We have here apparently a different instrument from the
embryotome, which we saw was a form of knife. This is
a pointed spike-shaped instrument. It must have had
much the shape of one of the huge bodkins in the Naples
Museum (Pl. LI, fig. 1).

Apparatus for fumigating the Uterus and Vagina.

Fumigation formed an important part of the treatment
of all varieties of disease of the uterus and vagina. The
notion that the uterus was an animal within the body
which could wander about on its own initiative and which
was attracted by pleasant smells and repelled by disagree-
able smells, was responsible for much of the treatment of
gynaecological diseases by the ancients. To make a fumi-

gation, Hippocrates directs us to take a vessel which holds about four gallons (δύο ἐκτέας), and fit a lid to it so that no vapour can escape from it.   Pierce a hole in the lid, and into this aperture force a reed about a cubit in length so that the vapour cannot escape along the outside of the reed. The cover is then fixed on the vessel with clay.   Dig a hole about two feet deep and sufficiently large to receive the vessel, and burn wood until the sides of the hole become very hot.   After this remove the wood and larger pieces of charcoal which have most flame, but leave the ashes and cinders.   When the vessel is placed in position, and the vapour begins to issue out, if it is too hot wait for some time; if, however, it be of the proper temperature the reed should be introduced into the uterine orifice and the fumigation made.   Oribasius, quoting Antyllus (*Coll.* X. xix) varies the treatment somewhat by placing a vessel similarly prepared underneath an obstetrical chair, which had an opening in the seat, allowing a leaden pipe connected with the tube of the fumigating vessel to be passed into the vagina.

A fumigating apparatus of a more portable nature is mentioned by Soranus (xxiii) who tells us that Strato, a pupil of Erasistratus, used to place in a small vessel of silver or bronze, closed by a cover of tin, herbs of various kinds, and, having adjusted a small tube to the vessel, the mouth of the tube was placed in the vagina, and the vessel was then gently heated.   Soranus admits that severe burning might follow this practice if unskilfully used.

Pessaries.

Greek, βάλανος, πεσσόν, πεσσός; Latin, *pessum, pessus, pessulum.*

Pessaries are frequently mentioned.   They are usually bags filled with medicaments and not mechanical supports. However, in ii. 824, Hippocrates says that prolapse of the womb is to be reduced and the half of a pomegranate is to be introduced into the vagina.   Soranus says that in prolapse Diocles was accustomed to introduce into the vagina a pomegranate soaked in vinegar.   He also says that a large ball of wool may be introduced after reduction, and Aetius, Oribasius, and Paul copy him.

Hippocrates (iii. 331) says that in cases of fistula in ano, after the introduction of a medicated plug of lint, a pessary of horn is to be inserted (βάλανον ἐνθεὶς κερατίνην).   This would appear to be partly to distend the rectum, but partly also most likely to carry medicament, like the leaden tubes full of medicaments which were inserted into the uterus.

A pessary of bronze was found in Pompeii (Pl. LI, fig. 2), and is described by Ceci.   It is hollow and has a plate per- forated with holes (evidently for stitching it on a band, to fix it round the body).   Heister figures a similar instrument.   It is impossible to say whether this specimen was intended for rectal or vaginal use.

CHAPTER X

SUTURES, ETC.

Sponge.

Greek, σπόγγος ; Latin, *spongia*.

Sponges were used for many purposes. Paul (VII. iii) says they should be fresh and still preserve the smell of the sea. They were applied with water, wine, or oxycrate to agglutinate wounds, and also soaked in asphalt and set fire to and applied to wounds to stop haemorrhage.

Galen (*De Simp.* xi) says he has seen haemorrhage stopped by applying a sponge dipped in asphalt to a bleeding wound and setting fire to it, and leaving the unburnt part to cover the wound. Celsus says a sponge dipped in oil and vinegar or cold water relieves gouty swellings. He also recommends a sponge dipped in vinegar or cold water for stopping haemorrhage.

Dioscorides says that fistulae may be dilated with sponge tents.

Scribonius Largus says that in epistaxis the nose may be plugged with sponge :

Proderit et spongeae particulam praesectam apte forfice ad amplitudinem et patorem narium figuratam inicere paulo pressius ex aceto per se (xlvi).

Soranus (xli) says haemorrhage from the uterus may be stopped with a sponge tent :

Ὁπότε τρυφερὸν καὶ καθαρὸν σπογγάριον ἐπιμήκες ὡσαύτως διάβροχον ὡς ἐσωτάτω παρεντιθέναι προσήκει.

Sutures.

Celsus (V. xxvi) says sutures should be of soft thread not overtwisted that they may be the more easy on the part :

'Ex acia molli non nimis torta quo mitius corpori insidat'.
They were made of flax. The apolinose described by
Hippocrates (iii. 132) is directed to be made of crude
flax (ὠμολίνου), the strands of which were stronger than
those of dressed lint. This also is what Paul used for the
deligation of arteries.

Galen alludes to sutures of wool, and Paulus Aegineta in
the operation for ectropion says :

'Afterwards we unite the divided parts with a needle
carrying a woollen thread, being satisfied with two sutures.'

We have no mention of catgut being used for this
purpose, though that substance was early known to the
Greeks. The Homeric harp was strung with catgut. In
fact χορδή, the term for harp-string, simply means intestines.
Paul used a woman's hair in a needle to transplant hairs in
trichiasis (VI. xiii). Horsehair was used to raise a pterygium in Paul VI. xviii, but it is not mentioned as being
used for suturing wounds.

Serres Fines.

Greek, ἀγκτήρ ; Latin, *fibula.*

Celsus (V. xxvi) in describing the closing of wounds
says :

Nam si plaga in molli parte est, sui debet, maximeque si
discissa auris ima est, vel imus nasus, vel frons, vel bucca,
vel palpebra, vel labrum, vel circa guttur cutis, vel venter.
Si vero in carne vulnus est hiatque, neque in unum orae
facile attrahuntur, sutura quidem aliena est ; imponendae
vero fibulae sunt ; ἀγκτῆρας Graeci nominant ; quae oras
paulum tamen contrahant, quo minus lata postea cicatrix
sit.

'Suture is indicated if the lesion is in a soft part, especially in the lobule of the ear, or the ala nasi, or the forehead,
or cheek, the edge of the eyelid, or the skin over the throat,
or the abdominal wall. But if the wound is in a muscular
part and gape, and the edges cannot easily be opposed, suture
is contraindicated, and fibulae (Graece ἀγκτῆρας) are to be used
in order that the cicatrix afterwards may not be wide.'

We have here contrasted two methods of closing a wound, and the conclusion is readily arrived at that sutures in the first case and some metal contrivance in the second are intended. Celsus goes on to say, however:

Utraque optima est ex acia molli, non nimis torta, quo mitius corpori insidat. Utraque neque nimis rara, neque nimis crebra iniicienda.

' Both are best made of soft thread, not too hard twisted that it may sit easier on the tissues, nor are too few nor too many of either of them to be put in.'

A consideration of various passages in which the Greek authors use the term leaves a distinct impression on one's mind that a metal clasp is intended. Thus Paul (VI. cvii), in treating of compound fractures, says that if a large portion of the bone is laid bare we use fibulae and sutures (ἀγκτῆρσι καὶ ῥαφαῖς). It must be confessed, however, that the words of Celsus render it difficult for us to assert with certainty that fibulae were metal clasps, and we find ancient commentators in equal difficulty. Fallopius and Fabricius d' Aquapendente think fibulae mean interrupted sutures. Guido de Cauliac thinks they mean metal clasps. There is just the possibility that a contrivance like our harelip pin with a figure of eight thread may be indicated. This would satisfy both sides of the question. If fibulae were metal clasps, however, we have several varieties of ancient fibulae that might have been used for closing wounds. That most suited for the purpose in hand seems to me to be one consisting of a small bar terminating in two hooks. Several of these from Roman London are in the Guildhall Museum (Pl. LII, figs. 5, 6, 7). They represent a useful form of 'clip' still in use by cyclists, and they could be applied to wounds to act on the principle of Malgaigne's hooks for the patella. A modicum of support for this view may be derived from the fact that whereas Galen, from whom the above passage on compound fractures is quoted by Paul, uses the word ἀγκτῆρσι, the codices of Paul almost unanimously have ἀγκίστροις. Fourteen out of fifteen give the latter rendering.

M 2

Band of Antyllus.

In the interesting dissertation which Oribasius gives on the subject of phlebotomy (*Med. Collect.* vii) he states that Antyllus directs us to apply a ligature of two fingers' breadth round the arm when going to let blood at the elbow. He says that they are mistaken who affirm that the same effect may be produced by applying the band below, for the veins will not then swell even if the arm be fomented. When going to bleed at the ankle the ligature is to be applied at the knee. When the blood does not flow well he advises us to slacken the bandage if too tight. This is the famous 'band of Antyllus'.

It is mentioned also in the pseudo-Hippocratic treatise on Ulcers (iii. 328) :

'When you have opened the vein and after you have let blood and have loosened the fillet (ταινίαν) and yet the blood does not stop.'

Paul also mentions the band, including one round the neck when the veins of the forehead are to be opened for ophthalmia. So far as we know the fillet was nothing more than a plain strip of linen or some such material, but Deneffe, commenting on two bronze fibulae which were found in the grave of the surgeon of Paris, conjectures that they may have been used to fix the fillet in venesection. I give figures of these after Deneffe, but it seems to me that these buckles are more likely to have belonged to the straps of a portable instrument-case of canvas or leather which had disappeared. One is a neat little heptagonal fibula, 2·8 cm. in its widest part, with a tongue 27 mm. long (Pl. LII, fig. 2). The other fibula is in the form of a penannular ring, formed by a two-headed serpent curved on itself so that the two heads look at each other, separated from each other by a space of a few millimetres (Pl. LII, fig. 8). Opposite the heads there is a small rectangular opening to receive the end of the strap. There is no tongue.

It may have been fixed by a metal bar attached to the other
end of the strap.

Sieves and Strainers.

Greek, ἠθμός, κυρτίς ; Latin, *cribrum.*

Scribonius Largus mentions sieves of different sizes. In
ch. xc a small one is mentioned :

Contunditur hic cortex per se et cribratur tenui cribro.

In other places larger sizes are mentioned :

In his macerantur res quae infra scriptae sunt, contusae
et percribratae grandioribus foraminibus cribri (cclxix).

Marcellus (*De Medicamentis,* xxxiii. 9) says :

Pulverem facito, et cribello medicinali omnem pulverem
cerne et permisce, et cum vino vetere calefacto locum inline.

There are large numbers of sieves and strainers in bronze
and earthenware in the Naples Museum.

Paul (VII. xx) says oil of sesame is to be prepared from
sesame pounded, softened, and pressed in a strainer with
screws (διὰ κυρτίδων τῶν κοχλιῶν). The word κυρτίς literally
means a basket or wicker eel-trap. Here it must mean a
strainer.

Mortar and Pestle.

Greek, ἰγδίον, mortar: δοῖδυξ, pestle ; Latin, *mortarium,
pilum.*

In the find of the oculist Severus is a bronze dish which
Deneffe regards as a mortar. It is 8 cm. in diameter and
3·5 deep, and rests on a base of 3 cm. diameter, so that it
sits firmly. Marcellus (*De Medic.* i) mentions a mortar of
marble :

Haec universa conteres in mortario marmoreo, et aceto
admixto fronti inlines.

He also mentions one of wood :

Huius radicem colliges et findes in partes duas, quarum
unam siccabis ac minutatim concides et mittes in pilam
ligneam atque illic diligenter tundes (xxiii).

Scrib. Larg. speaks of pestles of wood :

Hoc medicamentum cum componitur pilum ligneum sit (clii).

In Paul we have a mortar of lead and a leaden pestle mentioned several times :

'Εν μολυβδίνῳ ἰγδίῳ καὶ μολυβδίνῳ δοίδυκι λειώσας.

' Triturate ceruse with wine and rose oil in a leaden mortar with a leaden pestle and anoint with it' (III. lix).

Galen (*De Simpl.* x) speaks of bronze mortars :

' Wherefore, some call only the natural mineral by this name, but some also the substance which is prepared in a bronze mortar with a copper pestle by means of the urine of a boy, which some value according to the differences of the verdigris. But it is better to prepare it in summer, or at least in hot weather, rubbing up the urine in the mortar, and it answers the more excellently if the bronze of which you make the mortar is red and the pestle too, for more is thus rubbed off by the turning of the pestle when the bronze is of a softer nature.'

Paul mentions a mortar of marble. A small mortar of bronze was found amongst the instruments of the surgeon of Paris. Another small one from my own collection is shown in Pl. LII, fig. 3. The excavation of the temple of Aesculapius in the forum has brought to light a large number of mortars of marble. They are mostly about six or seven inches in diameter, but are much deeper in proportion than our modern mortars are. The spathomele and other olivary probes were no doubt often used as small pestles.

Whetstone.

Greek, ἀκόνη ; Latin, *cos.*

We saw that several of the slabs on which ointments were prepared had evidently been used for sharpening knives, and whetstones are often found of varying degrees of roughness from sandstone to fine argillaceous smooth stones. Paul (VII. iii) says :

Τό γε μὴν τῆς Ναξίας ἀκόνης ἀπότριμμα ψυκτικὸν εἶναι φασὶν ὥστε καὶ τιτθοὺς παρθένων καὶ παίδων ὄρχεις προστέλλειν. τῆς ἐλαιακόνης δὲ τὸ ἀπότριμμα ῥυπτικὸν ὑπάρχον ἀλωπεκίαις ἁρμόττει.

'The filings of the Naxian whetstone are said to be re-frigerant, repressing the breasts of maidens and the testicles of boys. The filings of the oilstone being detergent suit with alopecia.'

It is uncertain what the Naxian whetstone was, but it was considered the best variety of whetstone. It is men-tioned in Pindar. From the fact that emery is found in Naxos one might conclude that the Naxian whetstone was of emery, but a few lines before the passage quoted from Paul he has already mentioned the emery:

Ἡ δὲ σμύρις ῥυπτικὴν ἔχουσα δύναμιν ὀδόντας σμήχει.

'The emery having detergent powers cleanses teeth.'

Galen makes the Naxian stone a variety of ostracites which was apparently marble formed of shells. One of the marble ointment tablets had, we saw, been used as a whetstone, but the whetstones for which Naxos was famous must, if not emery, have been some variety of shale or slate. It seems contrasted to some extent with the 'oilstone', i. e. whetstone which required oil. This was a clay slate (see Pliny, H. N. xxxvi. 47).

There are several whetstones from Stabiae in the Naples Museum which are classed among surgical implements. Whetstones are common objects in the finds from any Roman settlement, but they are not ground to regular shapes as our whetstones are. They usually consist of fine sandy schistaceous shale.

CHAPTER XI

ÉTUI, ETC.

Portable Outfit.

AFTER describing the larger apparatus necessary for the equipment of the surgery, Hippocrates mentions a portable equipment for use on journeys:

' Have also another apparatus ready to hand for journeys, simply prepared, and handy too by method of arrangement, for one cannot overhaul everything' (i. 72).

The component parts of this portable outfit so far known to us are as follows:

The scalpels of different shapes seem to have been carried in boxes, probably wooden, which opened in two halves like a modern mathematical instrument box. In these the scalpels lay head and tail, separated from each other by small fixed partitions. A box of scalpels of this kind is represented in a marble votive tablet which was found on the Acropolis on the site of the Temple of Aesculapius. A similar box with different instruments is seen in a donarium in the Capitoline Museum. The probes and forceps were carried in cylindrical cases like those in which the scribes carried their pens. A good many of these have come down to us. From the fact that in the grave of the surgeon of Paris there were found two buckles, it is probable that there had been buried along with the instruments a case of leather or some such perishable material, which had been used to contain instruments, but which had disappeared when the grave was opened. There have also been found boxes of various shapes for containing medicaments, cylindrical boxes for drugs in sticks, boxes divided into little partitions for drugs in semi-solid form, and other boxes for powders.

Portable Probe Cases.

The spatulae, sounds, hooks, and forceps were carried about in a cylindrical case of bronze. Several of these étui have been found containing instruments. They average 18 cm. in length and 1·5 cm. in diameter. The lid lifts off. One in the museum at Lausanne was found in a Roman conduit at Bosséaz and contained a cyathiscomele of the usual type (Bonstetten, *Recueil des Antiqq. Suisses,* pl. xii, figs. 11 and 12). A case exactly similar to the above containing a cyathiscomele and a toothed vulsellum was found in the Rhine Valley. Another case of the same kind was found at Bregenz. It contained a long ligula, a spathomele, a cyathiscomele, and a double olivary probe.

In the Naples Museum are four of these cases, three of which were found in Pompeii and one in Herculaneum. One of these is a plain cylindrical case 18 cm. long and 1·5 in diameter. It contained instruments (Pl. LIII, fig. 1). Another case is ornamented with raised rings. It was found in the House of the Physician, and contained six specilla of different kinds and a vulsellum. A third is of similar size and shape, but it is considerably destroyed by oxidation, and it is adherent to a rectangular slab of black stone which had been used for mixing medicaments. Through the cracks in the case there may be seen the probes which it contains. The case from Herculaneum is a plain cylindrical case 19 cm. long and 2 cm. in diameter.

Lately, several other cases have been found in Italy which are placed in the Naples Museum. One in a fragmentary condition showing its contents is seen in Pl. LIII, fig. 2.

In the Musée de Cinquantenaire, Brussels, there is one of these cases which was brought by M. Ravenstein from Italy. It contained three instruments all of silver, a cyathiscomele, a grooved director, and a plain double-ended stylet. It is 18 cm. long and 1·5 in diameter.

A fragment of a similar case was found in the Roman Hospital at Baden.

Box for Scalpels.

Among the ruins of the Temple of Aesculapius on the top of the Acropolis at Athens there was found a marble donarium or votive tablet, which represents a box of scalpels flanked by a pair of bleeding-cups.

The box reminds one of a modern box for mathematical instruments, being divided into a top and bottom half, each of which contains instruments separated from each other by small blocks. There are three instruments in each half and they are arranged head and tail. Five are scalpels of different shapes; the sixth has a curved cutting instrument at one end and at the other a lithotomy scoop. The size of each half of the box is 9 × 18 cm. outside measurement, and 7 × 16·5 cm. inside. See Pl. IV.

A similar box is seen in a marble tablet in the Capitoline Museum at Rome. Here the instruments are different.

Ointment Boxes.

Among the instruments of the surgeon of Paris was a box which Deneffe regards as a portable unguentarium. Unlike the medicament boxes it is not divided into compartments and the lid lifts off instead of sliding in grooves. It is 83 mm. long, 45 wide, and 35 deep. A line running round the middle of the box divides it into two equal parts and shows the division between cover and box. On the top is a little ring attached by a little pyramidal eminence 1·5 cm. high by which the cover was lifted off. Several circular ointment boxes, some containing medicaments, are to be seen in the Naples Museum.

Collyrium Boxes.

A large number of cylindrical boxes containing sticks of medicament have been found in Pompeii. In the find of the oculist of Rheims there were five cylindrical boxes, all of the same size and shape. They were 14 cm. long and 12 mm. in diameter. The covers are 35 mm. high. In

them were the remains of sticks of collyria which they
had contained. The term collyrium includes in classical
writings not only liquid but also solid applications. Collyria
were often moulded into sticks for portability, and liquefied
with water, wine, white of egg, &c., as required. These boxes
which have come down to us are exactly similar to the case
shown in Pl. LIII, but they are on a smaller scale.

Slabs for preparation of Ointment.

In the Roman provinces small rectangular slabs are
occasionally found which have evidently been used for
rubbing medicaments upon. Some have also their edges
worn by the sharpening of scalpels. As they are rarely of
the stone of the country in which they are found they have
evidently been manufactured in Italy and carried by their
owners on their travels. They are rather rare. There are
two in the museum at Naples. One was discovered in
Herculaneum which is 13 cm. long and 8 cm. broad. A
cylindrical instrument case is adherent to it. The edges
are bevelled on its upper surface. One of similar size and
shape, but made of white marble, was found in the grave of
the surgeon of Paris. It shows by the hollowing out of one
of its edges that it has been used for sharpening scalpels.

There are two in the Archaeological Museum at Namur.
They are of black marble. They measure 11 cm. by 7·5, but
a bevelling of ·75 cm. all round reduced the top surface to
9·5 cm. by 6. One of these was found along with surgical
instruments in a second-century cemetery at Wancennes
near Namur.

There is one of a dark-coloured stone in the museum at
Chesters, Northumberland. A small specimen of my own
is shown in Pl. LII, fig. 4. Similar small slabs, engraved
with oculists' names and the names of drugs to serve as
seals, have been found in considerable numbers, but these
oculists' seals have already an extensive literature of their
own.

Boxes for Drugs.

A considerable number of medicament boxes have been
found. They are usually of bronze, rectangular and of
a convenient size and weight for carrying in the pocket. In
size they average 12 cm. in length by 7·5 in breadth and
2 in height. As a rule they are divided into four or more
small divisions by partitions. Those reported are as
follows :

There are two in the Royal Antiquarian Museum at
Berlin. Of these, one was found in the Rhenish country
between Neuss and Xanten. It is of bronze. Inlaid with
silver on its sliding cover is the figure of Aesculapius standing in a small temple.

The second, of similar construction and appearance, was
brought by Friedlander from Naples and presented by him
to the museum.

A third, in the museum at Mainz, was found in the Rhine
while dredging near the town. It is of bronze, 10 cm.
long, 8 wide, 2 in height. It weighs 123 grammes. The
sliding lid is decorated with the snake of Aesculapius,
twisted round the stem of a laurel tree. The tree and the
body of the snake are formed by inlaying copper in the
bronze. The outline of the head of the snake and the scales
of the body are of silver. On withdrawing the lid the
interior is seen to be divided into four compartments each
shut by a little hinged lid, which may be lifted by means
of a little ring. Two of these compartments are 6 cm. by 3,
the two others are 4 cm. by 3.

In the Naples Museum there are three of these boxes. They
are all of bronze and divided into compartments. One is
divided into five compartments. It is 18 cm. long by 8 wide
and 2 deep. Of the compartments three are 8 cm. by 2 and
two are 5 cm. by 3. There is at the upper end of the box
a small handle by which to carry it. Another box is 13 cm.
by 7·5. On removing the lid it is seen to be divided into
six compartments, two of which have hinged lids of their

own, like the Mainz box. These compartments still contain medicaments (Pl. LIV).

The third of the Naples boxes is of an unusual type. It is 12·5 cm. by 7·5, but it is 3 cm. high and is divided into an upper and a lower division each 1·5 cm. deep. Each division has a sliding lid of its own. The upper division is separated into four compartments, two of which are 7 cm. by 2 and two are 4 cm. by 2. The lower stage occupies the whole area of the box.

A medicament box of a unique character was in use in a chapel as a reliquary till its original use was pointed out. It is of ivory, and carved on its sliding lid is a representation of Aesculapius and his daughter Hygeia. Aesculapius carries in his left hand a staff, round which is coiled a snake, and in his right a pine cone. Hygeia carries a snake in her right hand, and in her left a bowl from which she feeds the snake. The execution of the design shows the box to belong to the third century. The box is divided into eleven compartments. It is now in the Castle Valeria at Sitten.

APPENDIX

I. INVENTORY OF CHIEF INSTRUMENTS IN VARIOUS MUSEUMS

ENGLISH MUSEUMS.

THE *British Museum* contains the following (Case ii. B) :

Bleeding cup (No. 2313) ; collyrium spoon with spout (two, Nos. 2314 –5); staphylagra (two, Nos. 2316–7); hook, sharp (No. 2318); ditto blunt, i.e. retractor (No. 2319) ; forceps (No. 2320) ; two-pronged retractors (Nos. 2322–6) ; scarifier (No. 2327) ; knife, steel (No. 2321); scalpel handles (Nos. 2331–9); spathomeles ; cyathiscomeles ; spatulae ; ligulae ; ear specilla ; aneurism needle (No. 2372); epilation forceps (narrow), ditto (broad), ditto ditto with catch.

The Guildhall Museum contains a good few instruments found in London, amongst others a considerable number of ear specilla, vulsella, lancets, and numberless instruments common to both domestic and surgical use, such as strigils, ligulae, styli, and needles. The Celtic cutting instruments are of interest for comparison. This collection is in many ways one of the most interesting we have in England.

The museum at Shrewsbury contains several surgical instruments from the ancient Roman city of Uriconium on which Wroxeter now stands. The most interesting is a bleeding lancet. There are also styli and an ointment slab and the seal of an oculist.

The museum at Chesters, Northumberland, containing finds from the Roman camps at Cilurnum, Procolitia, Borcovicus, and other sites on the Roman Wall, contains amongst other things hooks, spatulae, bougie, a triangular medicine weight of tin, forceps, needles of bone and bronze, borers, knife blades, ear specilla, steelyard, counterpoises, many in the form of snakes and therefore, perhaps, for pharmaceutical purposes, the serpent being the symbol of Aesculapius.

MUSEUMS IN FRANCE.

Saint-Germain-en-Laye. Outfit of Severus, viz. two iron pitchers, four bowls, mortar, two balances, seven forceps, one spathomele, scalpel handle, ditto damascened, spatulae (two), two knife-and-needle handles, four needle handles, olive-and-needle, scalpel-handle-and-borer, three sharp hooks, blunt and sharp hook, small blunt hook, seal. Also four scalpel handles, forty forceps, four pocket companions with forceps, fifty bodkins and needles, thirty-three ligulae, fourteen spathomeles, thirty cyathiscomeles, twelve olivary probes.

Le Puy-en-Velay. Outfit of Sollemnis, viz. two knife-handles, ditto damascened, amulet, fragments of two forceps, seal, spathomele.

Paris. Private museum of M. Tolouse. Instruments from the grave of the Surgeon of Paris—Large bronze bowl which contained:

1, Marble slab for preparing ointments; 2, amulet of black obsidian; 3, bronze ointment box with silver damascening; 4, 5, 6, 7, 8, five cylindrical boxes for collyrium sticks; 9, 10, two buckles; 11, pharyngeal insufflator; 12, collyrium spoon; 13, 14, 15, three spathomeles; 16, 17, probes; 18, polypus forceps and scoop; 19, 20, epilation forceps; 21, 22, vulsella (toothed); 23, staphylagra; 24, 25, coudé vulsella; 26, spathomele of elegant form; 27, bleeding cup; 28, three-pronged fork.

Louvre Museum. Double curette, cyathiscomele, ear probe, stylet with large olivary point, forceps with olivary point.

Cluniac Museum. Scoop probe, scalpel.

Orfila Museum. All from Herculaneum. Ligula, ear scoop, two raspatories, hook and scoop, scalpel, fork and hook, curette and hook, bodkin.

Montauban Museum. (Tarn-et-Garonne.) Large surgical needle, cyathiscomeles (four), spathomele (one), scoop and spatula (steel), epilation forceps (one), four ear specilla, round spatula, bistoury handle, all from Cosa.

Rouen. Four epilation forceps, one small forceps with locking arrangement, one forceps with narrow rounded legs, one fine-toothed forceps, twelve cyathiscomeles, three needles and bodkins, twenty styloid instruments, three ligulae.

Amiens. Round scalpel handle with spiral lines, one large epilation forceps, one spud and probe, one blunt hook, one styloid probe, two spathomeles, six cyathiscomeles.

MUSEUMS IN BELGIUM.

Namur. Find of Surgeon of Wancennes, including ointment slab (Deneffe).

Brussels. Mus. de Ravenstein *alias* Cinquantenaire. Étui with silver specilla brought from Italy by M. Ravenstein; three specilla; scalpels.

Charleroi. Fine bistoury.

MUSEUMS IN GERMANY.

Mainz (Germano-Roman Museum). Spatula-probe, medicine box, staphylagra, four bleeding-cups.

Frankfort (Historical Museum). Four epilation forceps with sliding catch, two ligulae.

Kiel. Forceps of silver.

Cologne. Chisel, two forceps, pestle, phlebotome.

MUSEUMS IN AUSTRIA.

Vienna. Staphylocaustus.

MUSEUMS IN GREECE.

Athens. Six knives (four from tomb in Milos, two from tomb in Tanagra); forceps and porte-caustic, large cup and chain (Tanagra); ex-voto tablet from Acropolis, representing box of scalpels and two cups, twenty-four spathomeles, one trivalve vaginal speculum.

MUSEUMS IN DENMARK.

Copenhagen (Thorwaldsen). Two epilation forceps, one ditto with leaf shaped ends and catch, three spoon probes, one spatula probe.

MUSEUMS IN SWITZERLAND.

The instruments from the Roman hospital at *Baden*, now in the Baden Museum, have already been summarized (page 22). Instruments in other museums in Switzerland are :

Basel Augst. (Augusta Rauracorum). Uvula forceps, probe, spoon-probe.

Avenches. Broken uvula forceps, two vulsella, spatula of bronze plated with silver, probes, needle.

Yverdon. Probes.

Bern. Two probes from Hermance, forceps and spatula probe from Tiefenau.

Lausanne. Spoon probe from Bosséaz and Allaz. Étui for probes, seal for medicament pots, vulsella.

Sierre. Four spoon probes, spatula probe, large needle.

Schaffhausen. Probe from Schleitheim.

Zürich (Landesmuseum). A. Fifteen specilla (spathomeles) all with a sharp-edged long and narrow spoon at one end and at the other an elongated knob; length 130–160 mm.; seven from Galgenbuck in Albisrieden, seven from Windisch, one from Upper Italy. B. Small bronze instrument probably for extracting weapons from wounds ; present length 110 mm. (Naples). C. Probably a spatula for applying plaster (Athens). D. Ear spoons (three) of bone, 80–130 mm. long (two from Rome, one from Athens). E. Small bronze spatula, 125 mm. (Athens). F. Similar one of bone, 110 mm. (Windisch). G. Rod pointed at both ends, 155 mm. long. (Zürich). H. Bronze rod with a depression 30 mm. long in the middle, 225 mm. long (Windisch).

MUSEUMS IN ITALY.

Naples. Bleeding-cups (fourteen), spoons with bone handles (two), lancet and spoon, shears (bronze), fleams (veterinary), cannulae for ascites (two), bone elevators (two), catheter (one male, one female), bone forceps, specula uteri, trivalve and quadrivalve, speculum ani, toothed forceps, cauteries (three), needles, tongue tie guard, enema tube, probes, whetstones, étui, scalpels, medicament boxes, balances, ointment slabs.

Rome, Capitoline Museum. Curved double olivary probe, four spathomeles, four cyathiscomeles, thirty-six forceps toothed and plain, bodkins (four) eight cm. in length, three ear specilla, four ascites tubes, large scalpel, votive tablet with box of instruments.

Rome, Lateran Museum. Votive tablet representing forceps and other instruments.

Milan. Many knife blades, two bodkins, spathomele, two ligulae, scoop and curette, olive and stylet.

II. BIBLIOGRAPHY

CHOULANT.—De rebus Pompeianis ad medicinam facientibus. Leipzig, 1823.

KUEHN.—De instrumentis chirurgicis veteribus cognitis et nuper effossis. Leipzig, 1823.

In 1846-7 Benedetto Vulpes made a series of communications to the Royal Academy of Archaeology at Herculaneum as follows :—

(1) Illustrazione di un forcipe Ercolanese a branche curve. (March 3, 1846.)

(2) Memoria concernente la interpretazione dell' uso di un forcipe Ercolanese di bronzo con le estremità delle branche a semi-cucchiai dentellati : la illustrazione di due cannelli di bronzo anche trovati in Ercolano, de' quali servivansi gli antichi per cavar l'acqua dall' addomine degl' idropici : l'indicamento di tre cannelli Pompejani di bronzo. (April 28, 1846.)

(3) Illustrazione degli specilli e di altri strumenti chirurgici affini trovati negli scavi di Ercolano e di Pompei. (September 15, 1846.)

(4) Descrizione dello speculum magnum matricis e dello speculum ani. (November 24, 1846.)

(5) Delle pinzette, degli ametti, degli aghi chirurgici e del tridente scavati en Ercolano e in Pompeii. (December 1, 1846.)

(6) Illustrazione degli strumenti chirurgici di ferro trovati in Ercolano e in Pompeii. (January 19, 1847.)

In March, 1846, Quaranta made a communication to the same Society entitled ' Osservazioni sopra un forcipe Pompeiano ', in which he expressed a different opinion from that held by Vulpes, and pointed out that the forceps described by the latter in his first communication was found in Pompeii. This is the famous forceps which is always referred to as the ' Pompeian Forceps '.

These valuable papers of Vulpes and Quaranta were published in vol. vii of the *Memorie della Regale Accademia Ercolanese di Archeologia.* These articles are profusely illustrated. In 1847 Vulpes gathered these papers together, and with some slight alterations published them under the title of ' Illustrazione di tutti gli instrumenti chirurgici scavati in Ercolano e in Pompeii '.

At the time when Vulpes wrote there were in the Museum among other things 45 probes of various kinds, upwards of 90 forceps, 13 bleeding-cups of bronze, and 16 scalpels.

VACHER.—Les instruments de chirurgie à Herculanum et Pompeï. (*Gazette Médicale*, 1867, xxii. pp. 491–94.)

SCOUTETTEN.—Histoire des instruments de chirurgie trouvés à Herculanum et à Pompeï. (*France Médicale*, Paris, 1867, xiv. p. 483.)

OVERBECK.—Pompeji, 1884, p. 461.

Museo Borbonico, Vol. xiv. Pl. 35, Vol. xv. Pl. 23.

CECI.—Piccoli bronzi del Museo Nazionale di Napoli.

NEUGEBAUER.—Warsaw Medical Transactions, 1882.

NEUGEBAUER.—Über Pincetten alter Völker. (Korrespondenzblatt der Deutschen Anthropologischen Gesellschaft, 1884, No. 11.)

HAESER.—Lehrbuch der Geschichte der Medicin, 1875, p. 499.

GUHL and KOHNER.—Life of the Greeks and Romans, 1862, p. 296.

MONACO.—Guide Général du Musée National de Naples. (Naples, 1900.)

MONACO.—Les monuments du Musée National de Naples.

MONACO.—Specimens of domestic articles from the Naples Museum (Naples, n.d.).

LINDENSCHMIDT.—Die Altertümer unserer heidnischen Vorzeit, Bd. iv. Heft iii.

Anzeiger für schweizerische Geschichte und Altertumskunde, Jahrgang 1857, No. 3.

ULRICH.—Jahrbücher des Vereins für Altertumsfreunde in den Rheinländen, xiv. 1849.

ULRICH.—Catalogue of the Collection of the Antiquarian Society of Zürich (now placed in the Landesmuseum). Pt. I. Roman and Pre-Roman, by R. Ulrich, Conservator. (Published by Ulrich & Co., 1890, p. 140, pl. 1037.)

BRUNNER.—Die Spuren der römischen Aerzte auf dem Boden der Schweiz. (Zürich, 1894.)

ANONYMOUS.—Un hôpital militaire romain. Zürich. (A sketchy pamphlet published as an advertisement by the town of Baden.)

Mitteilungen der Antiquarischen Gesellschaft, Zürich.—References of interest occur in the following volumes : vol. vii, Meyer, Geschichte der XI. und XXI. Legion ; vol. ix, Mommsen, Die Schweiz in römischer Zeit (15) ; vol. xii, Die römischen Ansiedelungen in der Ostschweiz (19. M. B.) ; vol. xiv, Bochat, Recherches sur les antiquités d'Yverdon ; vol. xvi, Römische Alterthümer aus Vindonissa ; Römische Ansiedelungen in der Ostschweiz, ii ; vol. xvi, Bursian, Aventicum Helvetiorum, Mosaikbild von Orbe.

TOLOUSE.—Recherches historiques et archéologiques sur divers points du vieux Paris (Mémoires de la Société Dunkerkoise pour l'encouragement des Sciences, des Lettres et des Arts, 1885).

HAESER.—Lehrbuch der Geschichte der Medicin, 1875.

FREIND.—History of Physick from the time of Galen to the beginning of the Sixteenth Century, 1725.

DAREMBERG.—Histoire des sciences médicales, 1870.

McKAY.—History of ancient Gynaecology, 1901.

LAMBROS.—Περὶ σικυῶν καὶ σικυάσεως παρὰ τοῖς ἀρχαίοις.   Athens, 1895. An exhaustive monograph with many illustrations of ancient cups.

I. INDEX OF SUBJECTS

II.   LATIN   INDEX

III. GREEK INDEX

PLATE I

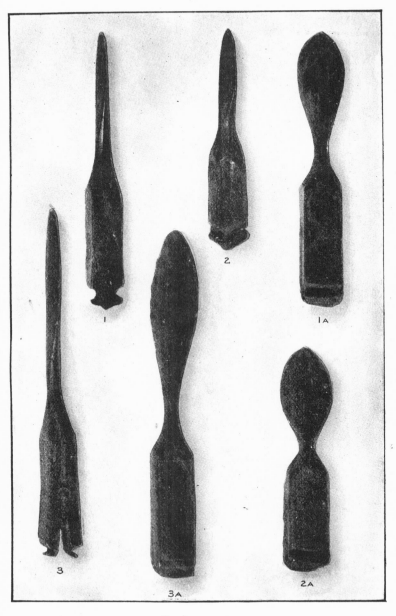

PLATE II

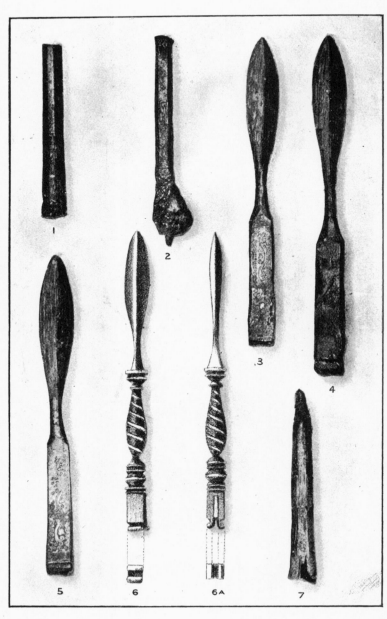

Size of originals.	Museum.	Size of originals.	Museum.
1. $5^{cm},2$	Saint-Germain	5. $10^{cm},5$	Saint-Germain
2. 6^{cm}	,,	6. $8^{cm},7$	Puy-en-Velay
3. 10^{cm}	,,	7. 6^{cm}	Saint-Germain
4. $11^{cm},5$	,,		

PLATE III

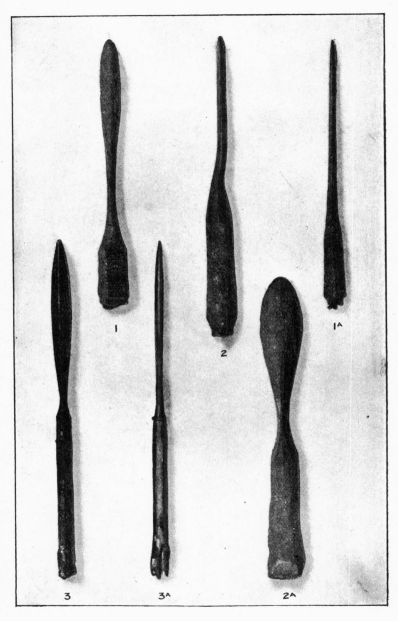

Size of originals.   *Museum.*

1. 7^{cm},5   British
2. 8^{cm},5   ,,
3. 12^{cm},2   Author's

PLATE IV

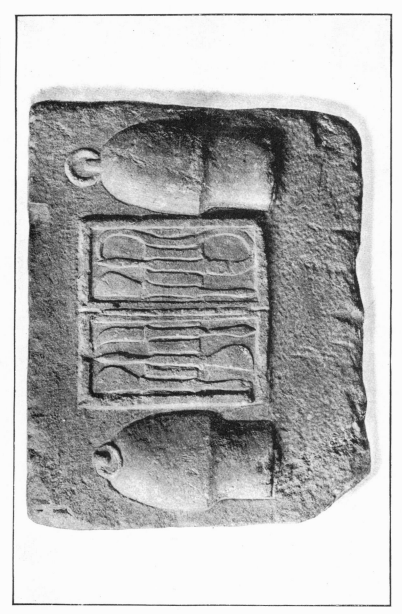

Museum.
Athens

PLATE V

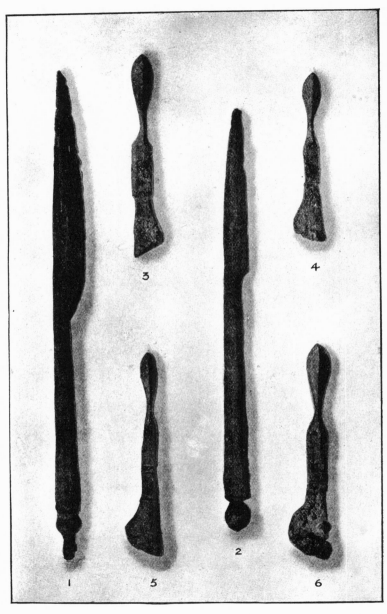

Size of originals.	Museum.	Size of originals.	Museum.
1. 14^{cm},3	British	4. 15^{cm},5	Naples
2. 12^{cm},3	,,	5. 17^{cm}	,,
3. 17^{cm}	Naples	6. 18^{cm}	,,

PLATE VI

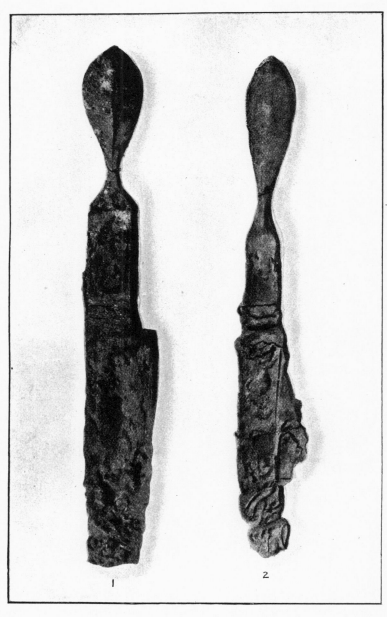

1

2

Size of originals.	*Museum.*
1. 15^{cm}	Naples
2. 14^{cm}	Charleroi

PLATE VII

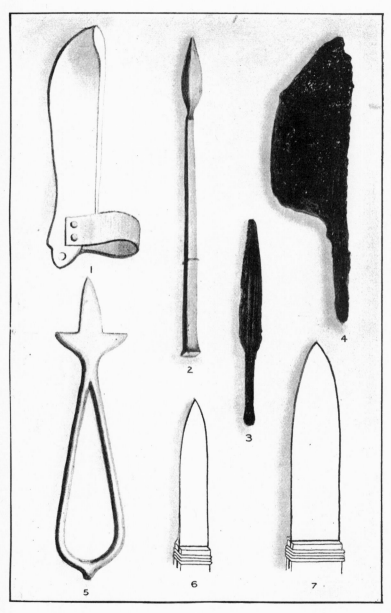

Size of originals.	Museum.	Size of originals.	Museum.
1.	Modern catalogue	4. 10ᶜᵐ,7	Author's
2. 9ᶜᵐ,5	Cologne	5. 11ᶜᵐ	Shrewsbury
3. 7ᶜᵐ,8	Author's	6, 7.	After Heister.

PLATE VIII

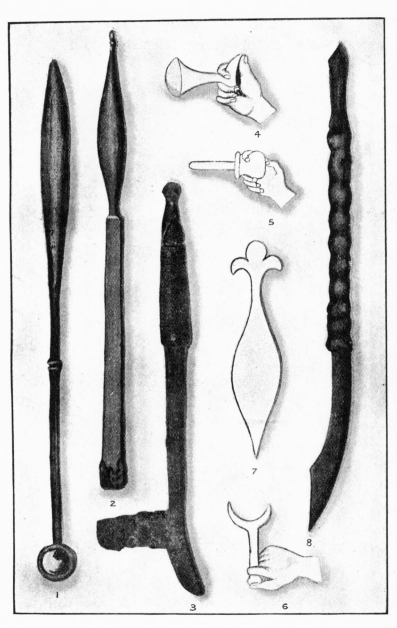

Size of originals.	Museum.	Size of originals.	Museum.
1. 15^{cm}	Montauban	4, 5, 6.	Hypothetical
2. 13^{cm},5	Bibliothèque Nationale	7.	After Albucasis
3. 12^{cm}	Naples	8. 14^{cm}	Orfila

PLATE IX

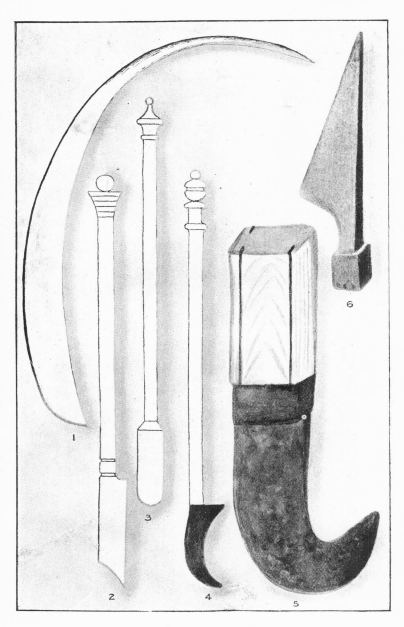

PLATE X

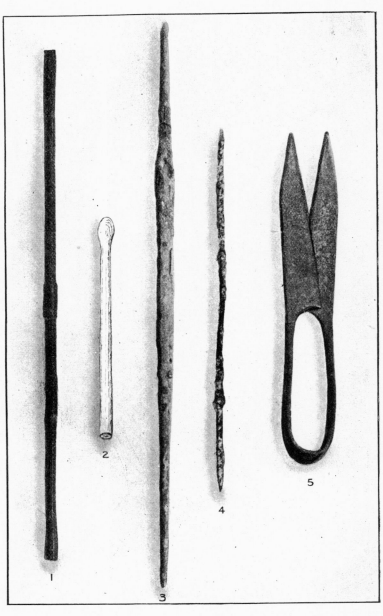

Size of originals.	Museum.	Size of originals.	Museum.
1. 15^{cm},7	Naples	4. 13^{cm},5	Author's
2. 6^{cm},5	Thorwaldsen	5. 10^{cm}	Naples
3. 17^{cm},6	Naples		

PLATE XI

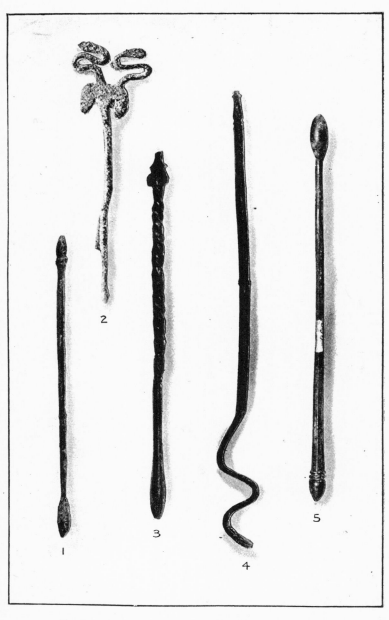

Size of originals.	Museum	Size of originals.	Museum.
1. 11cm,2	Author's	4. 18cm	Author's
2. 8cm	Baden	5. 12cm	Saint-Germain
3. 10cm,2	Author's		

PLATE XII

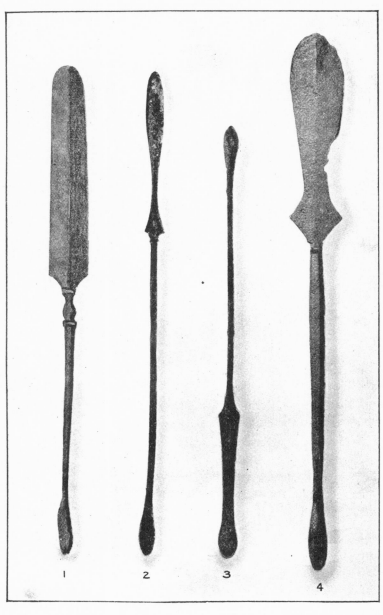

Size of originals.	Museum.	Size of originals.	Museum.
1. $14^{cm},5$	Naples	3. $17^{cm},2$	Author's
2. 18^{cm}	Author's	4. 18^{cm}	Athens

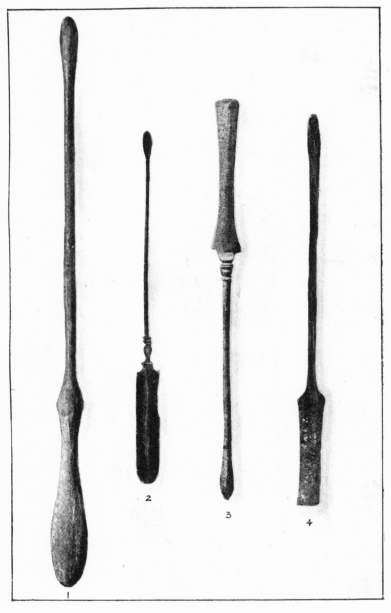

Plate XIII

Size of originals.	Museum.	Size of originals.	Museum.
1. 18cm,5	Naples	3. 17cm	Athens
2. 16cm	Mainz	4. 20cm	Author's

PLATE XIV

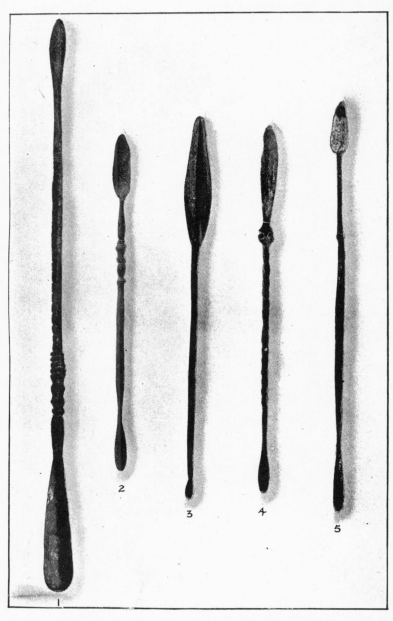

Size of originals.	Museum.	Size of originals.	Museum.
1. 17cm	Naples	4. 15cm,5	Mainz
2. 11cm	Author's	5. 12cm	Author's
3. 15cm,8	,,		

PLATE XV

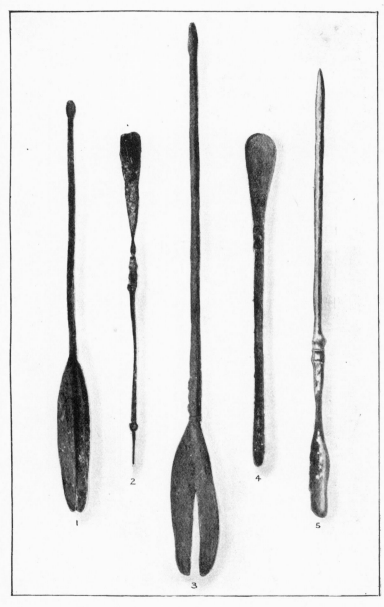

Size of originals.	Museum.	Size of originals.	Museum.
1. 17^{cm},2	Author's	4. 14^{cm}	Author's
2. 13^{cm}	,,	5. 13^{cm},8	Baden
3. 16^{cm}	Naples		

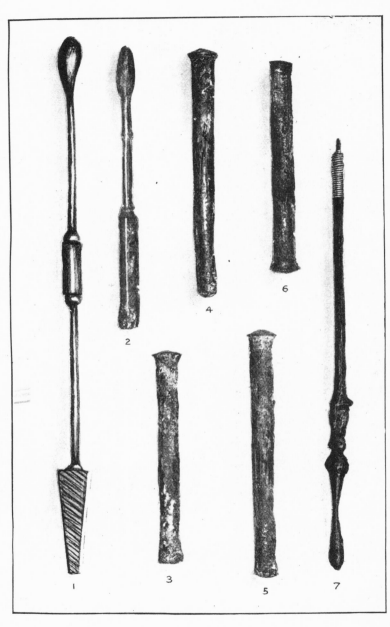

PLATE XVI

PLATE XVII

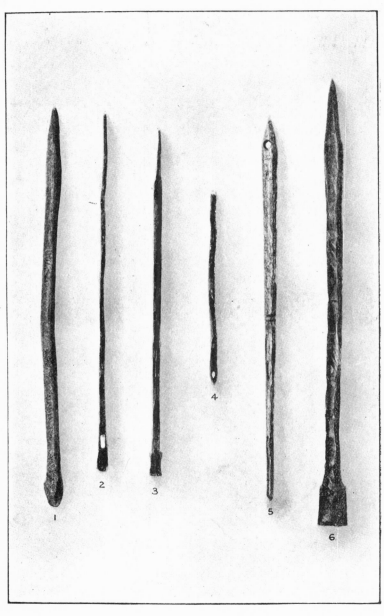

Size of originals.	Museum.	Size of originals.	Museum.
1. 11^{cm},5	Baden	4. 7^{cm}	Author's
2. 12^{cm},5	Author's	5. 10^{cm},5	,,
3. 14^{cm}	,,	6. 12^{cm},5	Naples

PLATE XVII

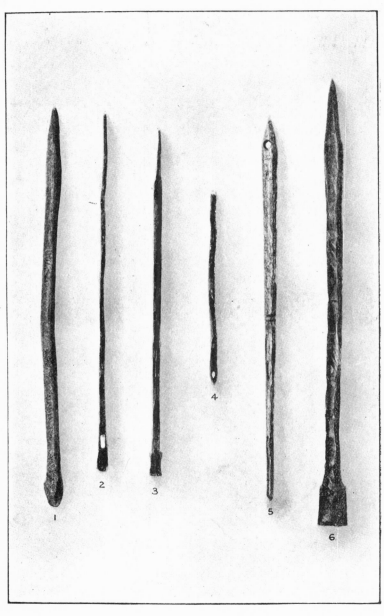

Size of originals.	Museum.	Size of originals.	Museum.
1. $11^{cm},5$	Baden	4. 7^{cm}	Author's
2. $12^{cm},5$	Author's	5. $10^{cm},5$	,,
3. 14^{cm}	,,	6. $12^{cm},5$	Naples

PLATE XVIII

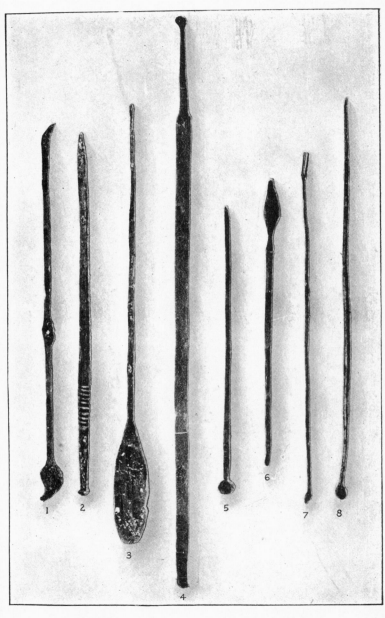

Size of originals.	Museum.	Size of originals.	Museum.
1. 11^{cm},2	Author's	5. 10^{cm},5	Author's
2. 10^{cm},8	,,	6. 10^{cm},5	,,
3. 18^{cm},4	,,	7. 14^{cm}	,,
4. 20^{cm}	,,	8. 16^{cm},7	,,

PLATE XIX

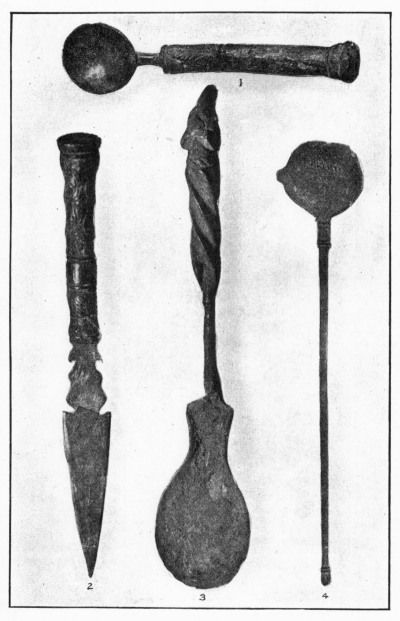

Size of originals.	Museum.	Size of originals.	Museum.
1. 7cm,8	Naples	3. 14cm,2	Naples
2. 12cm,2	,,	4. 17cm,5	British

PLATE XX

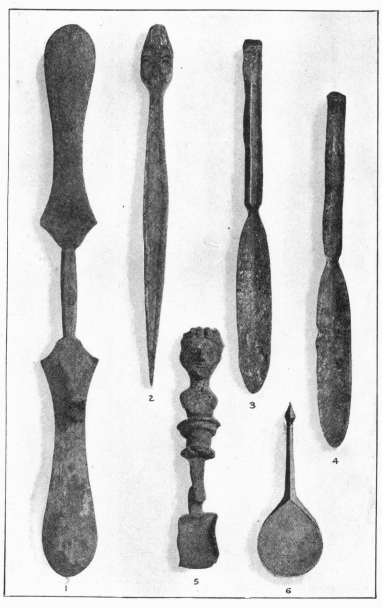

Size of originals.	Museum.	Size of originals.	Museum.
1. 17^{cm},5	Naples	4. 12^{cm}	Saint-Germain
2. 11^{cm},4	After Védrènes	5. 7^{cm},5	Naples
3. 12^{cm}	Saint-Germain	6. 11^{cm},5	After Védrènes

PLATE XXI

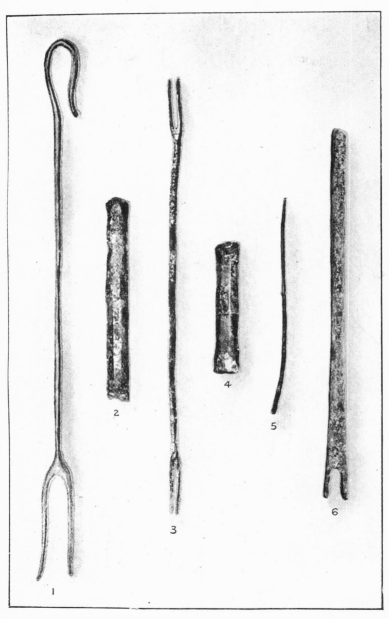

Size of originals.	Museum.	Size of originals.	Museum.
1. 15cm	After Védrènes	4. 4cm	Saint-Germain
2. 6cm	Saint-Germain	5. 8cm	Author's
3. 18cm,2	Author's	6. 10cm,2	,,

PLATE XXII

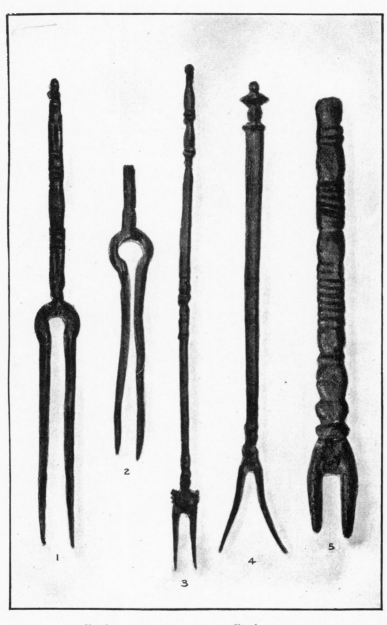

Size of originals.	Museum.	Size of originals.	Museum.
1. 12^{cm}	British	4. 14^{cm}	British
2. 7^{cm},5	,,	5. 10^{cm}	,,
3. 13^{cm},2	,,		

PLATE XXIII

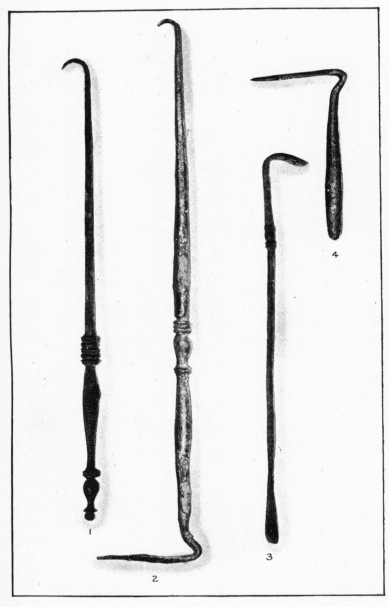

PLATE XXIV

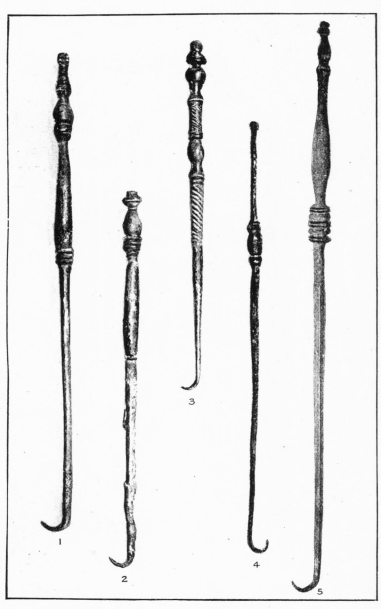

Size of originals.	Museum.	Size of originals.	Museum.
1. 14^{cm},8	Saint-Germain	4. 15^{cm},5	Author's
2. 11^{cm},5	,,	5. 17^{cm}	Naples
3. 10^{cm},8	,,		

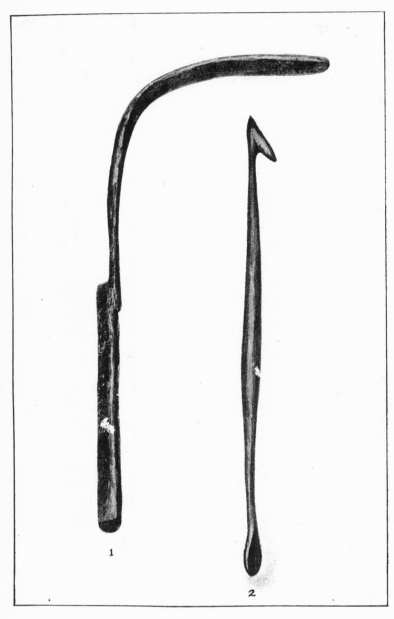

Size of originals.   *Museum.*

1. 21cm   Author's
2. 13cm,3   After Védrènes

PLATE XXVI

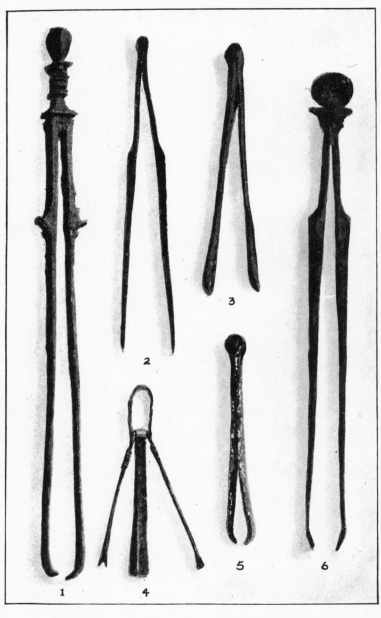

Size of originals.	Museum.	Size of originals.	Museum.
1. 17^{cm}	Naples	4. 6^{cm}	Guildhall
2. 9^{cm},5	Author's	5. 6^{cm},9	Author's
3. 8^{cm}	Naples	6. 15^{cm}	Naples

PLATE XXVII

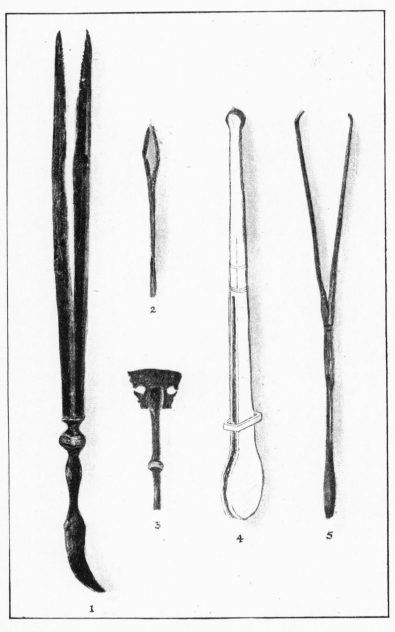

Size of originals.	Museum.	Size of originals.	Museum.
1. 15^{cm},5	Toulouse	4. 11^{cm},8	Thorwaldsen
2. 4^{cm},8	Saint-Germain	5. 11^{cm},8	Saint-Germain
3. 5^{cm},5	Mainz		

PLATE XXVIII

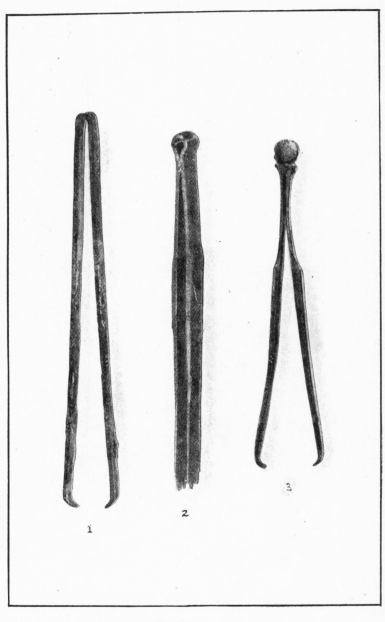

1

2

3

Size of
originals.   Museum.
1. 12ᶜᵐ,4   British
2. 10ᶜᵐ,5   Naples
3. 12ᶜᵐ   Author's

PLATE XXIX

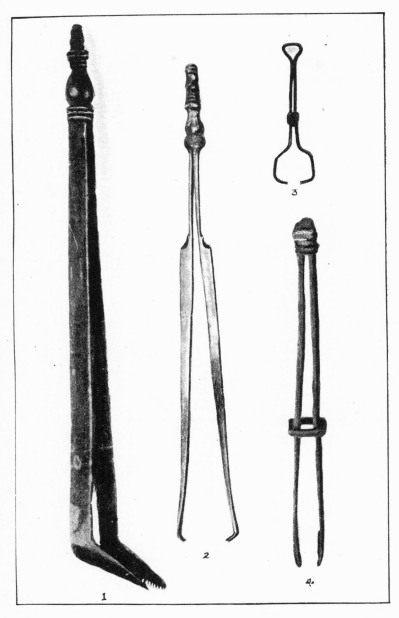

Size of originals.	Museum.	Size of originals.	Museum.
1. 17^{cm}	Toulouse	3. 5^{cm}	Mainz
2. 5^{cm},8	Saint-Germain	4. 10^{cm}	Naples

PLATE XXX

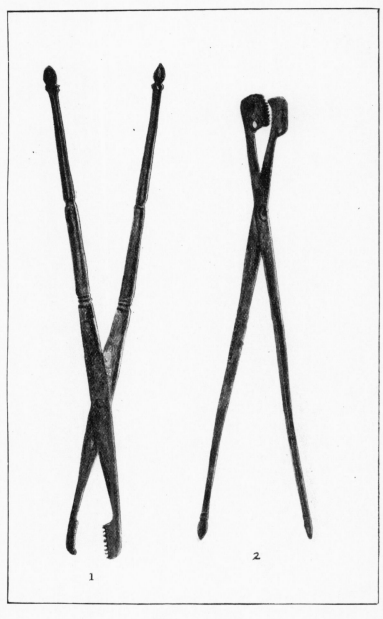

1

2

Size of
originals.   *Museum.*
1. 19^{cm}   British
2. 18^{cm}   ,,

PLATE XXX

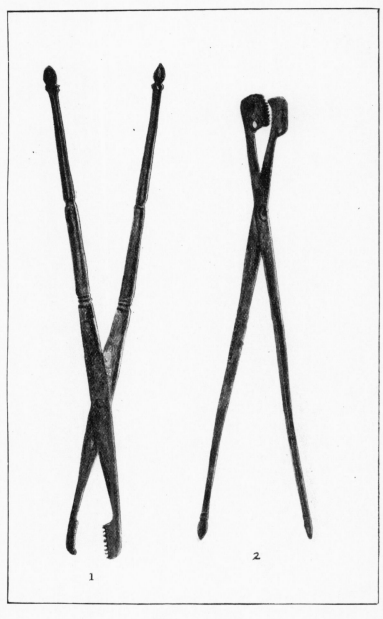

1

2

Size of
originals.   *Museum.*
1. 19cm   British
2. 18cm   ,,

PLATE XXXI

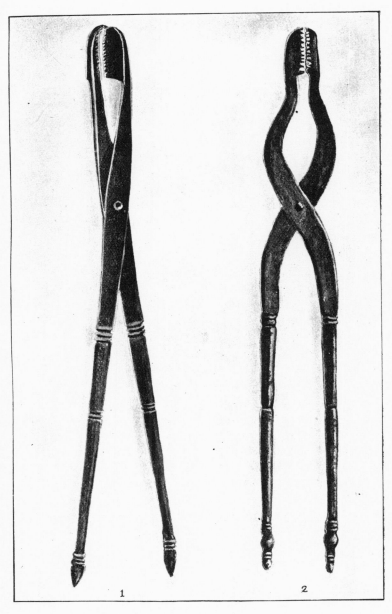

*Size of
originals.*   *Museum.*

1. 19^{cm}   Toulouse
2. 20^{cm},2   Basle

PLATE XXXII

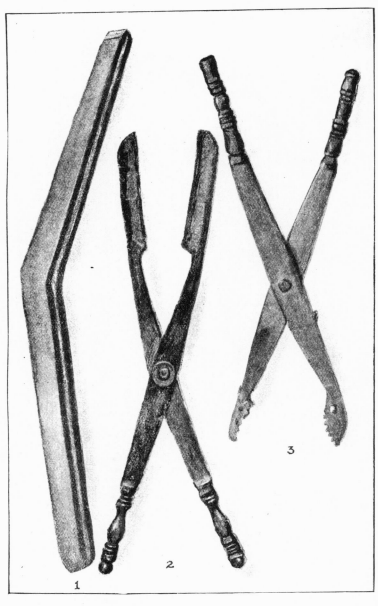

Size of originals.

1. 15^{cm},2
2. 12^{cm},5
3. 11^{cm}

Museum.

After Védrènes
Vienna
Naples

PLATE XXXIII

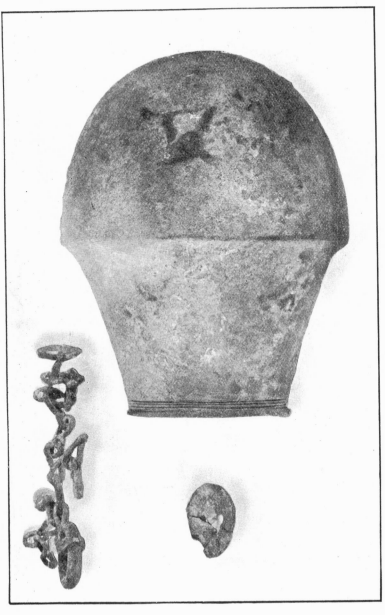

PLATE XXXIV

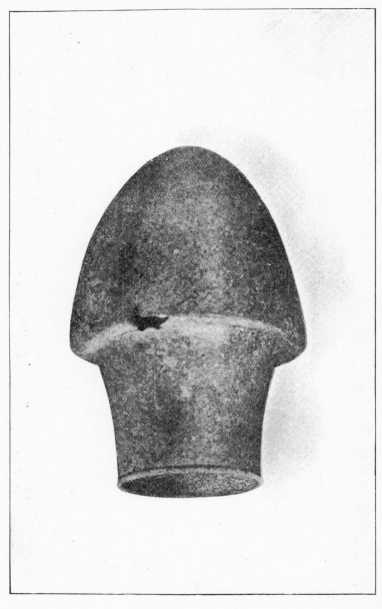

PLATE XXXV

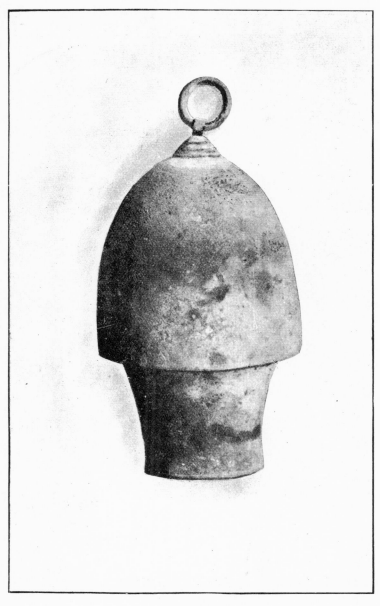

PLATE XXXVI

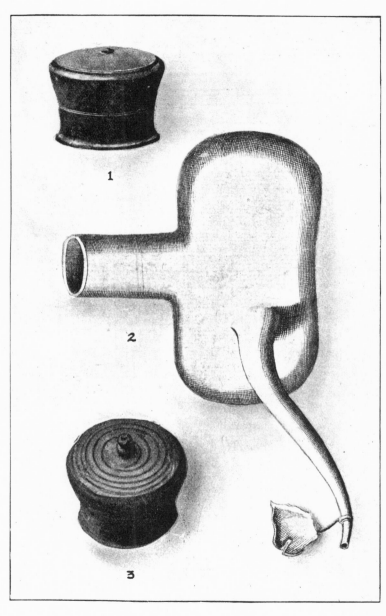

PLATE XXXVII

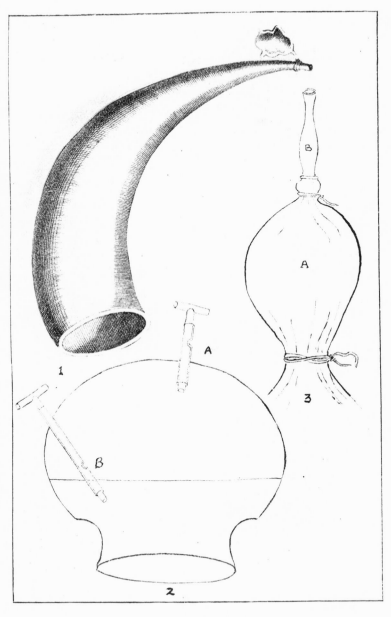

1. After Alpinus
2.   ,,   Hero
3.   ,,   Heister

PLATE XXXVIII

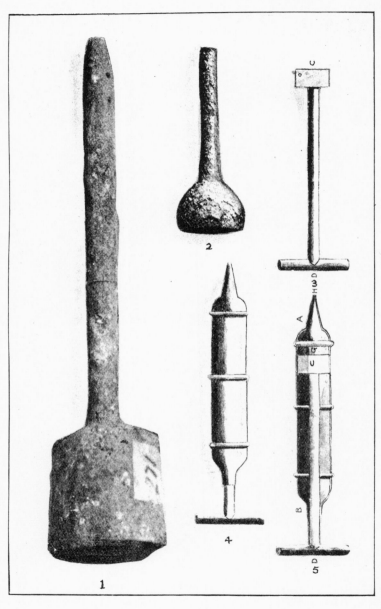

Size of
originals.

Museum.

1. 13^{cm}   Naples
2. 5^{cm},5   Baden
3, 4, 5.   After Hero

PLATE XXXIX

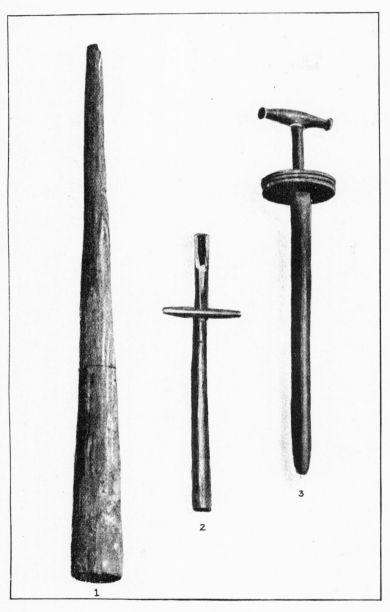

PLATE XL

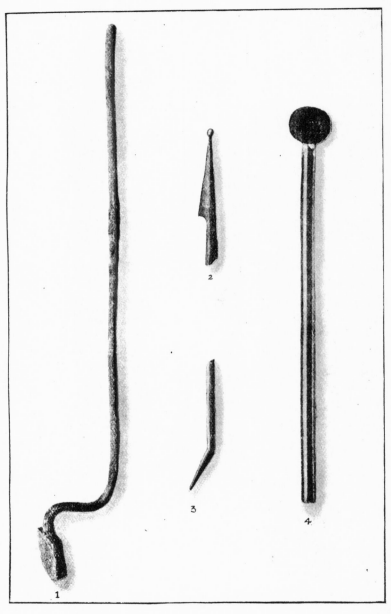

PLATE XLI

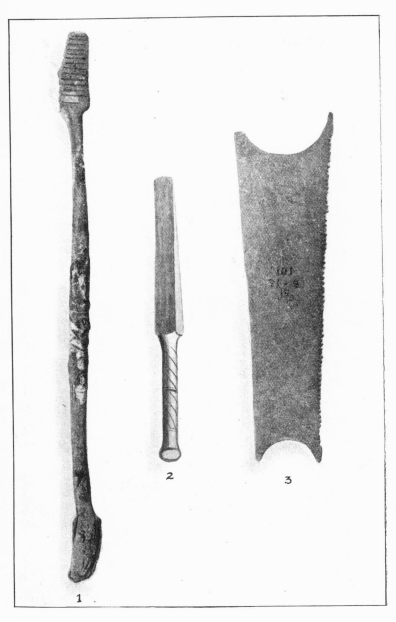

1

2

3

Size of originals.	Museum.
1. 15^{cm},5	Naples
2. 8^{cm},5	Cologne
3. 11^{cm}	British

PLATE XLII

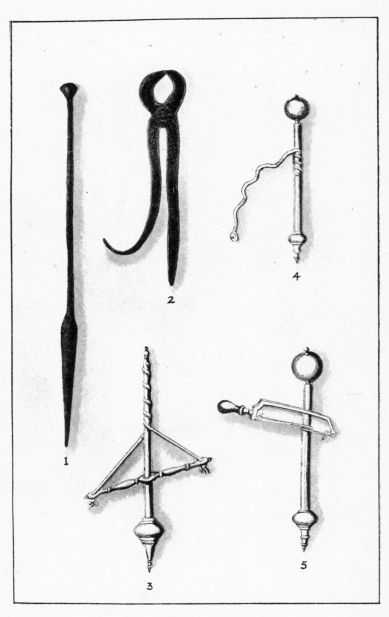

PLATE XLIII

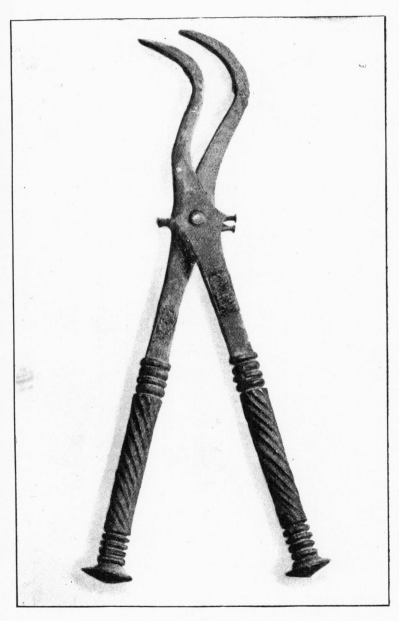

PLATE XLIV

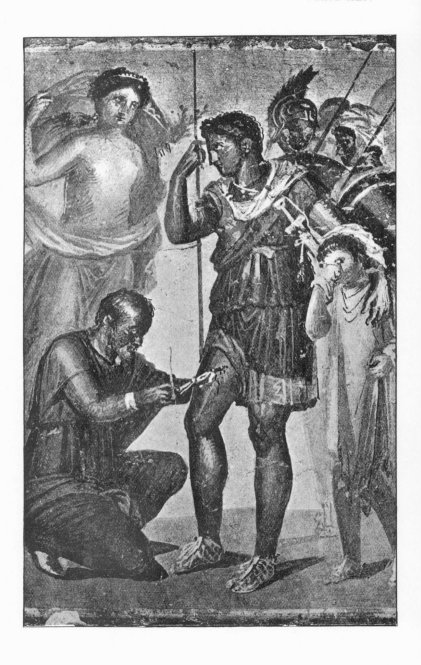

PLATE XLV

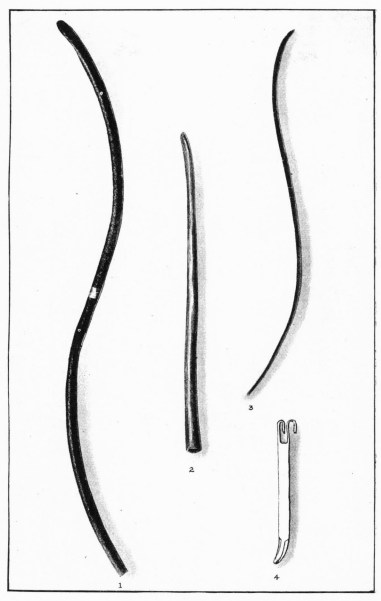

Size of originals.	Museum.	Size of originals.	Museum.
1. 26^{cm},5	Naples	3. 15^{cm}	Mainz
2. 20^{cm}	,,	4.	Hypothetical

PLATE XLVI

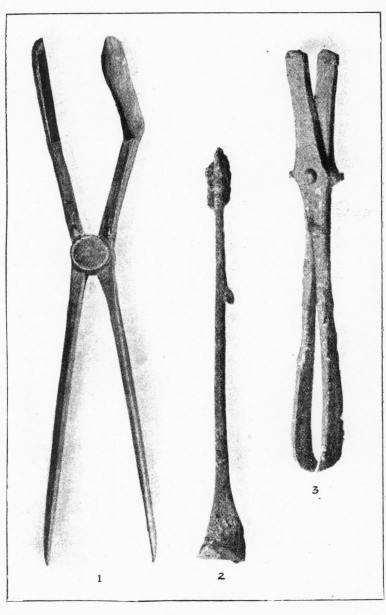

1

2

3

Size of originals.   *Museum.*

1. 15^{cm}   Naples
2. 11^{cm},5   ,,
3. 11^{cm},5   ,,

PLATE XLVII

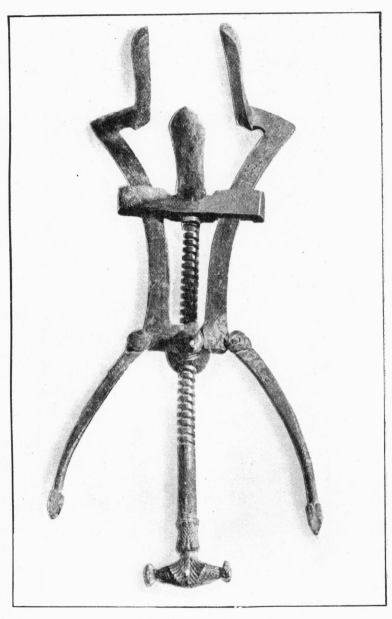

PLATE XLVIII

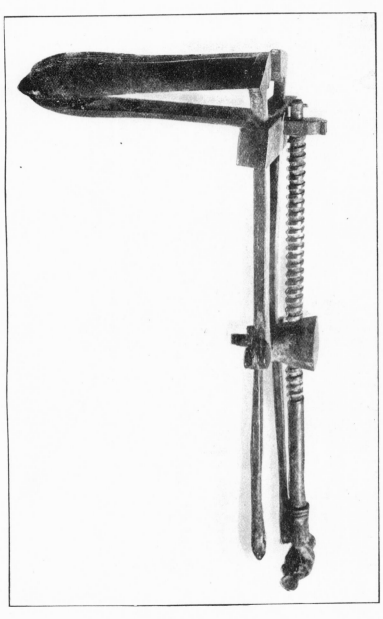

PLATE XLIX

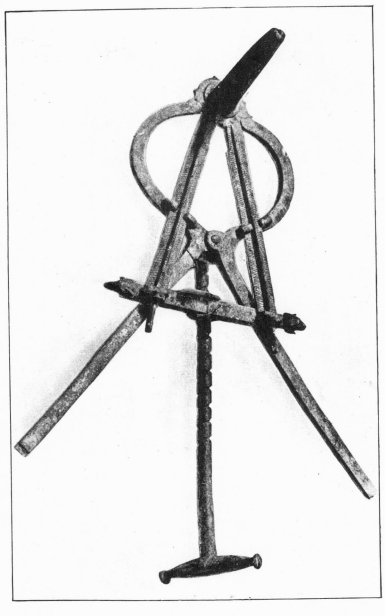

PLATE L

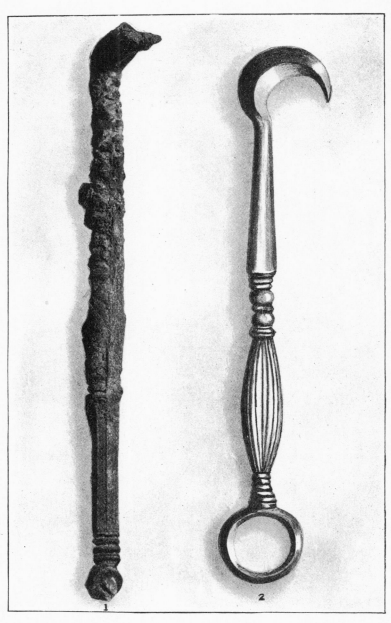

Size of
originals.   *Museum.*

1. 17^{cm}   Naples
2. 15^{cm},3   After Védrènes

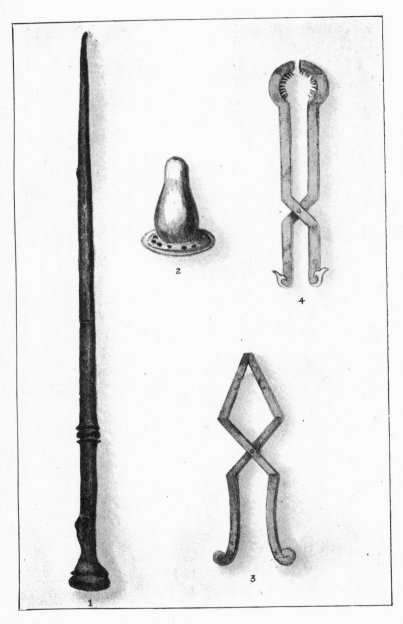

PLATE LI

PLATE LII

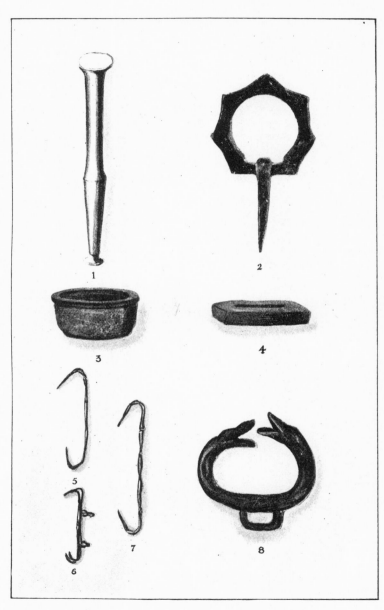

	Size of originals.	Museum.		Size of originals.	Museum.
1.	6^{cm}	Cologne	5.	5^{cm}	Guildhall
2.	3^{cm}	Toulouse	6.	4^{cm}	,,
3.	2^{cm} × 4^{cm},2	Author's	7.	7^{cm}	,,
4.	4^{cm},4 × 2^{cm},5	,,	8.	3^{cm},6	,,

PLATE LIII

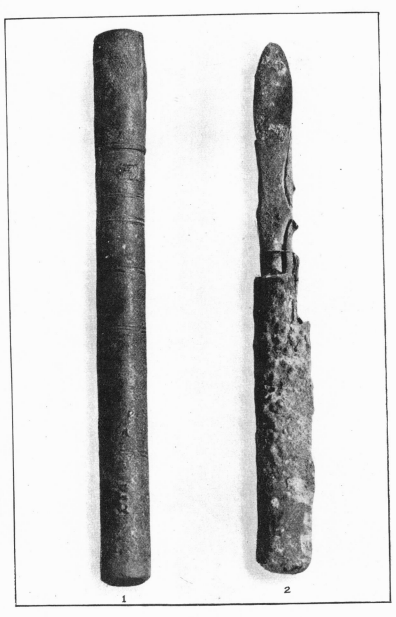

Size of originals.	Museum.
1. 18ᶜᵐ	Naples
2. 17ᶜᵐ	,,

PLATE LIV

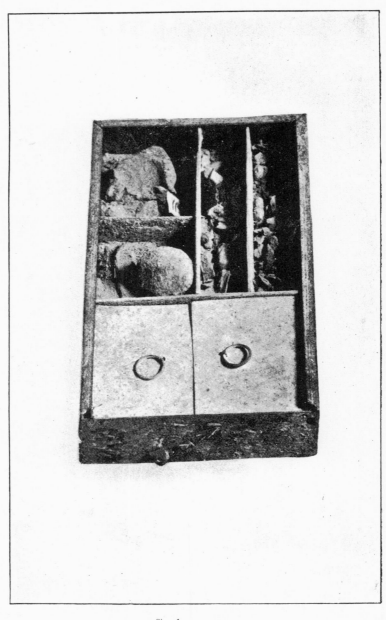

Size of
original. Museum.

13^{cm} × 7^{cm},5 Naples

DATE DUE

OCT 14 1991			
OCT 28 1991			
NOV 13 1991			
OCT 28 1996			
SEP 30 1996			
GAYLORD			PRINTED IN U.S.A.